YOUR PREGNANCY MONTH BY MONTH

OBSTETRICAL AND GYNECOLOGICAL GROUP

730 24th STREET, N.W.
WASHINGTON, D.C. 20037
202-338-8383

9801 GEORGIA AVENUE
SILVER SPRING, MD. 20902
301-681-5111 till 2 p.m.

AFTER 2 p.m. — WEEKENDS AND HOLIDAYS
CALL 202-338-8383

IF NO ANSWER — 301-206-1061

CLARK GILLESPIE, M.D.

YOUR PREGNANCY

MONTH BY MONTH

Third Edition

A Harper Colophon Book

1817

HARPER & ROW, PUBLISHERS, New York
Cambridge, Hagerstown, Philadelphia, San Francisco
London, Mexico City, São Paulo, Singapore, Sydney

YOUR PREGNANCY MONTH BY MONTH (*Third Edition*). Copyright © 1977, 1982, 1985 by Clark Gillespie, M.D. All rights reserved. Printed in the United States of America. No part of this book may be used or reproduced in any manner whatsoever without written permission except in the case of brief quotations embodied in critical articles and reviews. For information address Harper & Row, Publishers, Inc., 10 East 53rd Street, New York, N.Y. 10022. Published simultaneously in Canada by Fitzhenry & Whiteside Limited, Toronto.

Designer: C. Linda Dingler

Drawings by Patricia K. Tribell

Library of Congress Cataloging in Publication Data

Gillespie, Clark.
  Your pregnancy month by month.

  Includes index.
  1. Pregnancy. 2. Obstetrics—Popular works. I. Title.
  [DNLM: 1. Pregnancy—popular works. WQ 150 G478y]
  RG525.G513   1985   618.2   84-48601
  ISBN 0-06-181310-9   85 86 87 88 89 10 9 8 7 6 5 4 3 2 1
  ISBN 0-06-091257-X (pbk.)   89 10 9 8

*THIS BOOK IS DEDICATED WITH A GREAT
DEAL OF LOVE TO THE MANY
THOUSANDS OF WOMEN WHO HAVE
ENTRUSTED THEIR MOST VALUABLE
POSSESSIONS—THEIR LIVES AND THE
LIVES OF THEIR UNBORN BABIES—
TO MY CARE.*

CONTENTS

WHERE TO FIND
WHO AND WHAT

Telephones

Doctor's Office _____

    Home _____

    Exchange _____

Hospital _____

Pharmacy _____

My Mother _____

His Mother _____

Ambulance _____

Taxi _____

"Dial-a-Prayer" _____

Delicatessen _____

Travel Help

How to find a competent doctor in foreign countries:

    International Association for Medical Assistance to Travelers
    Empire State Building
    350 Fifth Avenue
    New York, New York 10001

(Fees for all IAMAT physician calls in foreign countries are standard.)

Advice on flying:

Airtransport Association of America
1709 New York Avenue, N.W.
Washington, D.C. 20006
(202) 626-4000

Pit stops for tired, hungry, thirsty, bladder-pressed drivers:

National Association of Truck Stop Operators
P.O. Box 1285
Alexandria, Virginia 22313
(703) 549-2100

Many of these stops have inns, shops, laundries, banks, etc., on a 24-hour basis.

INTRODUCTION

The first edition of this book was published in 1977. In the very few years that have elapsed since then, our society has witnessed, and indeed participated in, a quantum leap in obstetrical care. New technology, changes in laws, and changes in social and moral attitudes have so altered the childbearing environment that many situations and practices that were once accepted are now out of date and have been discarded—sometimes even before they are recorded. The cutting edge of change (and not all change is necessarily better!) moves rapidly.

Maternal mortality has declined 50 percent in the last ten years, and the *rate* of decline is increasing. Childbearing (but not child raising) is a safe procedure, and maternal death has all but disappeared as a factor in vital health statistics. It is actually now safer to be pregnant than it is to practice modern birth control—but that's a whole other story.

Having achieved a safe and favorable climate for pregnant women, physicians and scientists have been able to redirect more of their energies to the resolution and improvements of fetal well-being and survival. So it is, then, that the concept of a certain "right to be well born" has evolved. This right involves a triple-faceted covenant between the expectant mother, the physician, and society.

Physicians involved in maternity care are responsible for providing a level of obstetrical competence that is consistent with present and readily available knowledge—not what is on the horizon or in the papers, but what application and judgment say is correct for the times. Physicians must also clearly advise expectant mothers of their *own* responsibilities to provide the best internal environment for their babies.

And so, therefore, the expectant mother must comply with those needs of her unborn child of which she is aware and of which she has been made aware. She then will do her utmost to provide her growing and developing baby with the best she can. Many Americans live hazardously in the fast lane, and it seems virtually impossible to step off the track even when they are host to the sacred trust that is motherhood. No societal fad or fancy premise or practice, law or loophole can ever change that trust between mother and child; felt, suspected, or unfelt, it is there. So she must move to the outside lane and give it her best shot.

Society is obliged to yield to the needs of future generations. Unborn children are indirectly at constant and increasing risk from environmental pollutants of all sorts. Increasing background radiation, toxic working environments, polluted streams and rivers, toxic waste dumps, and on and on the malignant decaying list grows. Society must make water safe to drink, land safe to till, food safe to eat, air safe to breathe, so that the unborn child is protected and delivered into an environment in which it can live and flourish and enjoy and learn, in its own time, to nourish and protect future unborn generations.

Happily, society is beginning to address these problems. A good example is the formation of the Healthy Mother, Healthy Babies Coalition. This new and active group is made up of more than 250 physicians, nurses, health professionals, social workers, and other interested maternal and child health workers. They have established as a prime goal the reduction of infant mortality in the United States by at least 35 percent within the next five years. They are well on their way to achieving this goal and will be a positive societal force in the future.

It is within this framework that our triumvirate of doctors, women, and society provides all of us with the impetus to make your infant—all infants—healthy, God willing. Alas, it is not a perfect covenant; no human coalitions are. But it is a functioning, living, and positive covenant. We must all recognize and protect the matchless value of what is our own: our inheritance and our future.

A major goal of this book is to continue to help inform and lighten the burden of expectant mothers. An equally important goal is to contribute to the responsibility of the covenant. What this book tells you is not meant to replace your own doctor's help and advice. You must work together, since your doctor is a better and more personal source of information. This book only serves as supplemental assistance and provides an opportunity for you to record your own comments, questions, and events as your pregnancy unfolds.

Having a baby is serious business, no question about it. Moreover, it is just the beginning of a long trail of serious business that will occupy most of the rest of your life. But don't take it too seriously or you will miss the flowers along the way. That's good advice—the kind you don't generally get from your friends or family.

Never has there been a better time to have a baby. Godspeed and great expectations!

CHAPTER ONE

MY FIRST
LUNAR MONTH

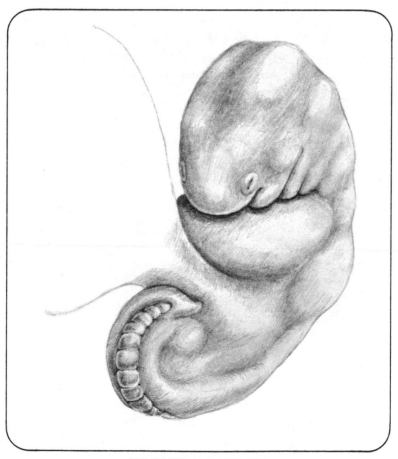

FIRST LUNAR MONTH

It's happened! A baby is on the way. Although you did not realize it, day 1 (or night 1)—the first day of your pregnancy and your baby's existence—has just slipped into eternity. Sometime during that twenty-four-hour period, conception occurred.

Your pregnancy began, of course, during the time of ovulation, about two weeks after the first day of the preceding menstrual period—which is confusing to some people and may be one reason (but not the main one) there are so many pregnancies.

Each month an egg is released from one ovary or the other by the process of ovulation, and it migrates into one of the two narrow fallopian tubes that lead to the uterus. There, if the egg comes in contact with sperm that have migrated up from the vagina, fertilization occurs. After fertilization the beginning embryo continues down into the uterus, or womb, where several days later it slips into a lush sugar-rich bed and there grows for some 265 days. The womb's inviting lining, having received and engulfed the embryo, remains intact in order to nourish it. Thus menstruation—the monthly shedding of the lining when it is not needed for a fertilized egg—does not occur. So the first and most common sign of pregnancy is the absence of menstruation.

The established pregnancy, new though it is, very soon exerts various changes upon you. These changes are initiated by certain cells that constitute part of the embryo. The very same cells are responsible for a positive pregnancy test. They also stimulate the pituitary gland to intense activity, and this gland in turn signals the rest of the body that really big things are coming.

A normal cyst, the corpus luteum, forms on your ovary at the point where ovulation occurred. This cyst lasts about three months then shrivels away. During its short lifetime, however, it is fundamentally important to the support of your pregnancy. It secretes the hormone progesterone, which under normal circumstances prevents you and your uterus from rejecting the pregnancy. Its function is taken over later by the growing placenta. Although this cyst is completely normal and necessary, it can cause some pain on whichever side it develops. Remember that.

The duration of pregnancy from ovulation to delivery averages 265 days—280 days from the first day of the last menstrual period. In this diary, day 1 is the day of conception, day 265 the expected date of confinement (EDC). Note, though, that only one woman in twenty delivers on this day; the vast majority deliver sometime within two weeks on either side of it. And some women hold on to their precious burden even longer. The longest recorded, thoroughly documented pregnancy was 340 days in duration! That's not likely to happen anymore, and we look with suspicion on pregnancies whose documented duration is over 42 weeks.

You can figure your expected date of confinement by adding seven days to the first day of your last menstrual period and counting back three months. Remember, though, that this is an *approximation*, and if you don't want your relatives and friends breathing down your neck at the bitter end, then neglect to announce your expected date—or add a few weeks to it. Otherwise there may well be a steady progression of telephone calls, visits and inquiries, secret conferences, and strange looks, all of which may cause you to wonder if you and your obstetrician know how to do simple arithmetic— particularly addition.

You will hear the term *lunar month* used in relation to pregnancy. A lunar month—a complete cycle of the moon—is 28 days. Since it is 280 days from the first day of the last menstrual period to the expected date of confinement, it is convenient to obstetrics to divide pregnancy into ten lunar months. It is convenient—but not shorter! Here in this book are ten chapters, one for each lunar month, and at the end of each chapter there is space for you to add your own thoughts and feelings and comments on events that took place during the lunar month—any medicine you took, any illness you had, nonemergency questions you wish to ask your doctor, and so forth. In such a way this book will become your personal diary of this pregnancy.

A very important thing to remember, regardless of what anyone may say—and this includes your friends, neighbors, both mothers, and all other people in important places and with big titles—is that pregnancy is not a disease and you are not ill simply because you are with child. Things can go wrong during pregnancy, and there may be a few bad moments and some abnormalities (and we will discuss most of them), but by and large you are not about to be consumed. At times you may find it hard to believe that a condition that consists of wake up, get up, throw up, fall out . . . (or, later on, when the only way to get out of bed is by rolling out . . . or it seems that you're pushing your burden instead of carrying it . . .) is not a dread disease; but it is not. And approximately 22,896,000 seconds after conception you will be delivered of the precious gift. That's more than anyone who is not pregnant can say.

Pregnancy Testing

From the dawn of time—or at least since humans became involved in it—the determination that a pregnancy actually exists has generated fantastic interest. You all know that. Pregnancies have launched and broken homes, launched and destroyed empires, launched and sunk a thousand ships. Pregnancies are generally of such enormous social, physiological, and emotional impact that the early determination of their existence has always engrossed human beings. In ancient cultures all manner of tests were devised to determine pregnancy. The saliva from a pregnant woman would supposedly make a goat throw up. A golden ring suspended over a woman's abdomen would spin wildly were she pregnant—in one direction if it was a boy, another if it was a girl. One hundred and fifty years ago the first urine pregnancy test was devised. After the urine lay flat on a plate for a few hours, it became covered with a misty, iridescent film, which sank to the bottom in five more days! And so on.

Modern medicine's romance with pregnancy testing began when it was determined that a substance secreted by the human embryo called human chorionic gonadotropin (HCG) began to circulate in maternal blood very early on. It was also established that this HCG was concentrated and excreted in maternal urine (but was not misty). This very specific hormone substance is secreted by embryonic cells almost from the moment of conception, and its secretion continues to increase, doubling every other day, reaching a peak at somewhere between days 60 and 80 of pregnancy and falling rapidly thereafter, but continuing to be secreted until delivery and for several weeks following.

Since HCG is concentrated in maternal urine, early pregnancy testing was carried out on concentrated urine samples. In fact, most office tests and all home pregnancy tests still are based on that principle. In the beginning, maternal urine was injected into rabbits and then frogs in order for HCG to stimulate activity in their reproductive glands. These tests were time consuming, expensive, not uniformly accurate, and very hard on rabbits and frogs! Today's chemical tests on urine are considerably more accurate, particularly if the urine is concentrated. The tests are based on a compliment fixation procedure that is somewhat complicated to explain, but we'll try. The test is prepared as follows: In the laboratory red blood cells are coated with the antigen HCG. These cells will now clump together when and if the antibody to HCG is added to them— unless that antibody is inactivated by some other HCG antigen. And that's where pregnant urine comes in—it has HCG in it. Thus when it is added to the other agents, the red blood cells will not clump and so the test is positive for pregnancy. If clumping occurs, the test is negative and pregnancy does not exist, or the urine specimen did not contain enough HCG antigen to neutralize (it was too early in the pregnancy, or the urine was too dilute).

Blood pregnancy tests, on the other hand, involve a radioimmunoassay process that measures very accurately the presence of HCG in maternal blood serum. Such tests are often positive a few days after conception, but usually their accuracy is not dependable until shortly after the first missed period.

Beta HCG

This blood pregnancy test is the most valuable diagnostic pregnancy test available today. Beta HCG is one tiny spectrum of the whole HCG complex, and it is *very* specific for pregnancy. If there are greater than three units of beta HCG in the maternal serum, pregnancy exists or has very recently existed. Our knowledge of beta HCG can help us do the following:

- Establish a very early, reliable diagnosis of pregnancy.
- Determine pregnancy health. As we have already noted, the beta subunit fraction should double every other day along with the full HCG spectrum for the first 60 to 80 days, and as long as this is so, the pregnancy is generally healthy. If beta HCG stops doubling, we consider that something has happened to the fetus within the uterus or, of equal importance, the pregnancy may be abnormally located somewhere outside the uterus. Therefore, it is of value in following high-risk, abortion-prone pregnancies and also in helping to determine the presence of an ectopic pregnancy and the activity within such a pregnancy.
- Diagnose a very rare condition in which the placental cells have become abnormal and highly active and may even have induced a very rare cancer. This pregnancy test can follow

10

the course of such a placental abnormality and/or cancer and evaluate the treatment. Fortunately, this rare tumor, which once was uniformly fatal, now responds to new antitumor agents.

So we see that there are a variety of pregnancy tests available for use today at home, at the doctor's office, and in the hospital. And there are a number of social and medical reasons for knowing at an early date whether pregnancy exists. Let's look at some examples:

- The absolute diagnosis of pregnancy is particularly important in the case of someone with irregular menstrual periods who is having some symptoms of trouble, such as spotting or pain, or if it is suspected that the pregnancy may be outside the uterus.
- Diagnosis is important in high-risk pregnancies. The very sensitive beta-HCG pregnancy test is used to follow high-risk pregnancies in which there is a history of repeated abortions, to follow pregnancies in which there is a problem such as spotting or cramping, to determine for certain whether a fetus is living or dead, and to determine the outcome of ectopic pregnancies, as we will see.
- It is essential to have a test result as early as possible if a therapeutic abortion is being contemplated. The sooner the diagnosis is made, the simpler the abortion.
- It is also of importance to have the diagnosis confirmed if distant or prolonged travel is being contemplated.
- Since certain drugs and certain X-ray examinations could interfere with or damage a pregnancy in the early stages, pregnancy should be confirmed. Elective surgery, too, should be avoided.
- A teacher in a school where a rubella (German measles) epidemic breaks out should know if she is pregnant so she can get away from that environment as soon as possible, unless she is immune to the disease.

There are other compelling reasons to test, including just the burning desire to know. And so the pregnancy test is a very common procedure.

In summary, urine pregnancy tests available today are usually performed on a morning specimen (because it is the most concentrated) and take just a few moments to a few hours to interpret. Generally, these tests are not accurate until about two weeks after the date of your first missed period—between the third and fourth week of pregnancy. If the test is obtained from *well-concentrated* urine and if it is positive, then it is virtually 100 percent correct. If it is negative, a repeat test a few days later may be in order, unless your menstrual history is very unreliable. Two negative pregnancy tests, using good concentrated specimens of urine, provide fairly conclusive proof that a living pregnancy does not exist. These facts hold for both office and home urine pregnancy tests. Finally, blood pregnancy tests using radioactive immunoassay methods are now being used widely and can confirm pregnancy accurately a few days after the first missed period—and sometimes even before that landmark event.

Your Doctor

Selecting Your Doctor

There are some very important matters you should consider in choosing a doctor. Do you want a doctor with a single, partner, or multiple practice? Many obstetricians practice in groups of varying sizes. In this situation you may not see the same doctor on each prenatal visit or see the doctor you prefer as often as you want. Outweighing this is the fact that twenty-four hours each day and night at least one member of this group is available. He or she knows you, has your records, and is ready to serve you.

If you are thinking of prepared childbirth, will your doctor go along with it? Or, for that matter, does he or she share your feelings about bonding, parenting, and sibling training? Is your doctor's hospital convenient for you? Will your baby be able to room in with you? And be sure to find out if both the hospital and your obstretrician allow the father's presence in the labor and delivery room, even if you're having a cesarean section.

Most physicians practicing obstetrics now have special training, and there are two certifying bodies in the United States. One is the American College of Obstetricians and Gynecologists; another is the American Board of Obstetricians and Gynecologists. Both require examination in order to qualify a physician for membership, and the American College offers a great number of excellent postgraduate courses for obstetricians.

"Oh, for the good old days of the family doctor," you say, the doctor who did anything and everything and could always be called upon. Yes, and also in those same good old days there were leeches for bleeding the ill; turpentine enemas for typhoid fever; newspapers, boiling water, whiskey, and biting bullets for the delivery room. You forget there were a lot of sick mothers in the good old days and, sadly, a lot of dead mothers. Besides, you are more liberated than women in earlier generations, and your relationship with your doctor is not as dependent as theirs. The idea now is to have a warm, meaningful, one-to-one relationship. Essentially your obstetrician provides you with a service that makes you feel secure, not with a crutch. It is a better and a more satisfying relationship than the old dependent one. Doctors are not perfect, nor has anyone else been in the last two thousand years; that is just our human experience and condition.

Calling Your Doctor

Once you have selected and met your doctor, get to know him or her, the staff, the office hours, and what to expect from the answering service. You will do well to know in advance what telephone numbers to dial days, nights, weekends, and holidays. Most doctors list both their home and their office phone numbers in the telephone book. Instead of the home number, you may find the number of the physicians' exchange, which is a professional answering service able to locate your doctor twenty-four hours a day. In the very unlikely event that you can't trace your doctor in an emergency, go to the hospital you have selected. The staff there will do the looking for you, and most likely there will be someone at the hospital to take care of you until your doctor arrives.

While we're at it, let's set down a list of principles to apply when you call your doctor.

- If at all possible, call your doctor during office hours. Your records are at the office, as is a staff of trained personnel who can answer many of your questions. It does not make it any easier for you or your doctor if you call after office hours, when your doctor is "not so busy."
- When you reach the doctor's office, identify yourself, say that you are pregnant, tell your due date and when you last visited the office. When you are with the obstetrician you may be made to feel that you are the only patient that exists, but this obviously is not so. It therefore helps, particularly if you have to call at night, for you to present this information.
- Your mate, except for Saturday-night parties, is not a good historian of your obstetrical problems, and it wastes everyone's time for him to transmit questions back and forth over the telephone. So *you* talk to the doctor *yourself.*
- Don't leave a call for your doctor and go out of the house or, still worse, call someone for a little chat. Doctors may

14

take some time before calling you back, but remember, when you yourself are in the office talking about *your* problems, you don't like telephone interruptions to destroy the doctor's concentration on *you!*

- Know the phone number of the drugstore you prefer to use.
- Have a pencil and paper handy beside the phone when you make your call.

Last Menstrual Period

When you're having your first dialogue with your obstetrician or an associate, the number-one question will be: When was your last menstrual period? It would be to your advantage to have this information at the ready when you arrive for the first appointment.

Some women keep no such record, preferring instead to relate their last menstrual period to a local social event, political castastrophe, football game, or some other major landmark in their or others' lives. Your doctor doesn't have your frame of reference, and it is sometimes asking a lot for him or her to remember an event that is important to you. Therefore, do not tell the doctor that your last menstrual period was just before the Delta Epsilon door-to-door campaign for used Cabbage Patch dolls! Some well-organized women keep their menstrual information readily at hand on their checkbook, weekly diary, a grocery stub, bingo card, or some other meaningful data bank, well hidden in the recesses of their purse. But if you have no record, try to remember when your last menstrual period was before your next visit to your doctor.

Telling the Expectant Father

You don't have to faint nowadays to let your mate know that you are pregnant. In fact, most of the time there is no need to tell him anything—he already knows. After all, if he comes home night after night and finds you asleep, or if he finds that you spend all your waking hours in the bathroom, tending to one end or the other, he should be able to figure out that something unusual is going on, which should be enough to provoke some active curiosity around most young American households. Even more if it's an *old* household!

As our story unfolds, we will draw the expectant father more and more into the relationship that we hope you will develop with him during your pregnancy. We will talk about his relationship with you and with your doctor, about various educational classes and experiences that are now available in order to make a husband more of a participant who feels needed and wanted in the whole process.

Incidentally, a recent study showed that fully 60 percent of all expectant fathers had some symptoms of pregnancy; this is called the couvade syndrome. These poor men may have nausea and vomiting in the mornings, unusual food cravings, headaches, weight increases, and the like. Strangely, some animal fathers develop the same problems!

Sex Determination

Will it be Adam or Eve? Probably no other question is asked of an obstetrician more frequently than what the sex of an unborn baby will be. And yet a doctor's guess is just as good as and no better than yours. Without special tests, such as amniocentesis, chorion sampling, or sophisticated ultrasound, no one can predict the sex of an unborn child.

Of course, the sex is determined at the moment of conception. The mature female egg contains one sex chromosome, called X. The male sperm has a fifty-fifty chance of containing either an X or a Y chromosome. If an X-bearing sperm unites with an ovum, the child is a girl; if a Y, it's a boy. It is settled. Since the determination of the sex is dependent upon which sperm by chance fertilizes the egg, the sex of the child is therefore finally and forever determined by the male. Please note, though, that the *basic* embryonic plan of all mammals of both sexes is apparently feminine. Male development is due to an *interruption* of this basic plan! Think about that, ladies.

Can we *make* it a boy or a girl? This question is asked about as often as what sex is to be expected. If you wish to dip into folklore for a moment (and we will from time to time in this book), through all history there have been many attempts to preselect and predetermine the sex of an offspring. The only failure-proof folk method for controlling the sex of newborns was to destroy the sex not desired! As cruel as this may seem, various cultures, ranging from the Eskimos in the north to the Maori of New Zealand and the Toda of India, did exactly that. The result was nine living male births for every living female birth!

Such unacceptable procedures have long since vanished from the earth, it is to be hoped, and have been replaced by innumerable folk methods of attempting to select a child's sex at or before conception: certain chants to be recited during intercourse (not "Bolero"); timing of sexual contact in relation to wind direction, rainfall, temperature, phases of the moon or tides; eating sweet food to produce girls and bitter food to produce boys (which may have some relation to the old "sugar and spice and everything nice" rhyme). In the United States in years gone by, a man hung his pants on the right side of the bed if he wanted a son and on the left if he wanted a daughter—and put them away, I guess, if he just wanted to spend the night. However, this is not a very reliable method of planning the sex distribution of your family.

In fertility study centers, methods of sperm separation are being improved upon all the time, and we will eventually be offered mechanically or chemically separated X and Y sperm. Such sperm are being used in artificial insemination and in advanced fertilization centers where fertilization is accomplished outside the uterus and the fertilized embryo is then implanted in the womb.

Once your child is conceived, its sex can be accurately determined, as you already know, by a chromosome culture of amniotic fluid or, eventually, by chorionic sampling (see Appendix).

Here are some other unusual variations of the sex ratio at birth that may interest you.

- The percentage of male births is slightly greater than female.
- The percentage of male births rises during and after wars.
- The percentage of female births increases directly with the age of the mother, father, or both.
- The percentage of female births increases with birth rank— that is, first births are more likely to be male than are subsequent births.
- A higher percentage of sons is born to couples of a higher socioeconomic status.
- The ratio of sons to daughters is higher for couples with higher sexual intercourse rates.
- The ratio of sons to daughters is slightly lower among blacks than among Caucasians.
- Sex ratio varies with the seasons; in the United States, for instance, the ratio of male to female births is highest in June.
- The ratio of male to female births has been lower after certain natural disasters, such as floods, earthquakes, and epidemics.

Pills, Powders, and Panaceas

Our culture is pill oriented; we seem to have a pill for everything, from looking or feeling bad to smelling bad. Pills are adult pacifiers pushed by the pharmaceutical industry, huckstered by the communicators and gobbled by the billions.

This phenomenon is problem enough on its own, but thrust upon the pregnant community, it can become a nightmare in terms of its effect on two people: the host mother and the dependent, developing fetus. Studies show that pregnant women take an average of eleven over-the-counter drugs during pregnancy—the consequences of which are still largely unknown.

Before the thalidomide crisis, the safety of drugs prescribed for pregnant women did not have to be proved. Consequently, little was known in that area. Certain facts, however, are now clear from recent research. Almost any drug ingested by a pregnant women for whatever reason reaches the bloodstream of her child, in a proportional dose *equal* to or *greater* than hers and within a relatively short period of time. This period of time varies from drug to drug, and the relative concentration also varies to a certain extent. Generally speaking, it was once considered that the larger the molecular structure of a drug, the longer it took to cross the placenta and the less drug would be present on the baby's side. However, the so-called placental barrier can now be considered simply a myth. If you take a drug of any kind for whatever reason, it gets into your bloodstream and it almost invariably ends up in your baby's bloodstream as well. Some drugs actually *concentrate* on the fetal side of the circulation system. In other words, there is more drug present per ounce of baby's blood than there is per ounce of mother's blood.

Babies develop their organ systems and body structure almost completely during the first twelve weeks of pregnancy. At the end of that time they are very miniature but completely formed humans. For the remaining twenty-eight weeks of their gestation, these organ systems simply mature and increase in size. Therefore, the most critical period for producing structural abnormalities in the developing fetus is during the first twelve weeks. Further, deleterious drugs and diseases work their effects in varying organ systems depending upon when the drug is taken or when the disease is contracted. Using thalidomide as an example, if the drug was taken on the twenty-second day of the pregnancy, it produced disorders of the upper extremities; on the twenty-eighth day, disorders of the lower extremities.

It is important to realize that although development of the organ systems and body structure is generally completed by the twelfth week, there are some drugs and conditions that can affect the developing infant at various stages of pregnancy. The lack of proper nourishment, sudden and significant deficits in oxygen, certain types of radiation, and certain maternal habits such as excessive smoking, drinking of alcohol, work or drug addiction—all these and many others can harm your unborn baby at any period during pregnancy. These situations are discussed in other sections of this book.

I have in my office a vast accumulation of recent literature concerning drugs that can affect mothers and babies during pregnancy. It is not only vast; it is ominous and it is growing, for as you may already know, even "take two aspirins" is no longer considered a safe order. As far as self-medication is concerned, such simple and commonly used medications as aspirins, baking soda, and some cold preparations are not considered entirely safe insofar as harmful fetal effects are concerned.

As our story unfolds, we will be discussing in greater detail the effects of nicotine, alcohol, marijuana, LSD, heroin, and other drugs on the human fetus and on pregnancy. We will see what drugs obstetricians must use during pregnancy, labor, and delivery that may affect you and your baby adversely. And finally we will list what other medications, received from whatever source, are contraindicated in pregnancy. Today there are many drugs that are being used frequently as antidepressants, anticonvulsants, diuretics, antibiotics, and pain relievers that may have adverse effects on the human fetus. All these will be mentioned in their place.

What must be weighed and considered by you and your doctor first is the benefit-to-risk ratio that applies when using various medications during *your* pregnancy. *You* must remember never to use any medication without consulting your physician.

You must be aware of the effects of nicotine, alcohol, and other social drugs upon your pregnancy and, therefore, upon your baby, and make your own judgment as to their continued use. For the moment, it is reasonable to say that no drug given in the first weeks of pregnancy can be considered safe. Second, some women are employed in fields in which certain drugs, chemicals, vapors, or radioactive elements are present that make retirement from work a necessary consideration as soon as pregnancy is determined. This is covered on page 54.

What is important for you to remember, then, is that you take no medication during your pregnancy that is not prescribed by your doctor. Make sure you make any other physician you consult for any reason aware, if it is not obvious, that you are pregnant, and your obstetrician must concur in any treatment or medications given to you.

"Do As I Say"

We don't talk to each other that way anymore. Maybe we talk to some of our "little citizens" that way, but not to each other. Nevertheless, compliance ("do as I say") is, in medicine, a sensitive and vastly important subject that we need to talk about right now.

Many studies indicate clearly that medicines prescribed by physicians are not taken by their patients and that instructions they give are not regularly followed. This failure to comply with what we have been told and what we know is right involves all aspects of our lives (the use of seatbelts and baby seats in automobiles, for instance) and involves all of us, doctors included. We all know that. Now, when we are dealing with ourselves alone, compliance with medical instructions is a personal matter that each of us can deal with at a personal level, taking or disregarding what advice has been presented to us. Pregnancy is another matter—a loaded matter. For we are now dealing with the health and welfare of a helpless, dependent, and very, very vulnerable human being. So—give your baby your best shot. Follow your doctor's advice.

Ectopic Pregnancy

Whenever pregnancy occurs in an organ or location outside the uterus it is termed ectopic. Although this condition would seem to be very unusual, in actuality, the incidence of ectopic pregnancy is increasing, so that 1 percent of all pregnancies come to rest in an abnormal location. One reason for this increase is the exploding incidence of sexually transmitted pelvic infections in young women. Most frequently, the pregnancy sets up residence in one fallopian tube or another, but ectopic pregnancies are also found in the ovaries and even free in the abdomen. The most unlikely pregnancy of all occurs when the uterus and tubes have been surgically removed by hysterectomy. Under such strange circumstances we have to assume that a tiny sinus tract persists in the back of the vagina leading to the intraabdominal cavity, and it is through this that the sperm may migrate and actually fertilize an egg from ovaries that were left behind after the hysterectomy. Yes, ovaries left in after a hysterectomy may continue to ovulate; their resultant eggs ordinarily are absorbed without difficulty, just as they are after tubes are tied to produce sterilization.

Anyway, we are not fully aware of all the circumstances that can lead to ectopic pregnancies. They are certainly more commonly associated with acute and chronic pelvic infections, previous abdominal surgery, endometriosis, previous ectopics, repeated elective abortions, the use of IUDs, and other less common circumstances.

Usually ectopic pregnancies end within the first month or two after they have embedded, but the medical literature reports rare cases of pregnancies in the tube, in the ovary, and even in the abdominal cavity that have actually gone to full term and even survived.

The symptoms of an ectopic are those of pregnancy, coupled generally with pain in the region where it is embedded. Occasionally the pregnancy, being contained in a sac that cannot expand as can the uterus, suddenly ruptures. This produces a very acute condition accompanied by severe pain, intraabdominal bleeding, shock, and collapse. You should be suspicious of such an abnormal pregnancy occurring if you are overdue, have persistent lower abdominal cramping of a menstrual character (more likely on one side), and episodes of weakness or occasional vaginal spotting.

Thus if a fertilized egg implants in, say, the left fallopian tube, then besides the usual signs of pregnancy (missed periods, tender breasts, etc.), there will be increasing left-sided cramping pain. Note, though, that many other conditions of early *normal* pregnancy produce side pains of varying degrees, ligament pain and corpus luteum pain being two good examples. So don't panic—but call your doctor.

Generally the treatment of an ectopic pregnancy is surgical removal upon establishment of the diagnosis by your physician. This is not a dangerous operation unless, of course, the pregnancy has ruptured the containing area and there has been a great deal of bleeding and shock to accompany the rupture.

Although the risk of a recurrent ectopic pregnancy is just around 10 percent, nevertheless the chances of later having a *normal* term pregnancy are reduced by considerably more than that figure as revealed by present-day statistics. Again, the reason for this is uncertain.

It is important that an early diagnosis be made of an ectopic pregnancy whenever possible. This is not simple to do, but physicians are being assisted by the new beta HCG pregnancy test and by more sophisticated ultrasound procedures and other diagnostic techniques (see Appendix). Moreover, when an early diagnosis is made and confirmed, it is sometimes possible, by newer surgical methods, to save the affected fallopian tube so that it can function again in the future. Not all maternity centers are as yet fully equipped to do this, but the trend in that direction is encouraging.

Avoid!

This book is written from a positive point of view, with stress put upon what you can do rather than on what you cannot. But there are some things you need to avoid. Let's get it said now.

- *Any drug for whatever reason* unless cleared by the doctor responsible for you during your pregnancy. This includes over-the-counter nonprescription drugs—even aspirin. Record in this book any drug that you may have taken inadvertently before your pregnancy was diagnosed.
- Violent physical activity. Exercise and sports are fine, as you shall see, but exhausting, stressful physical competition directs more blood to skeletal muscles to sustain performance. Thus visceral organ centers are deprived of blood—and this includes the uterus. Abortion or damage is therefore more likely.
- Smoking.
- Alcohol. Should be ingested sparingly (1 ounce per day) or not at all.
- Certain paints. (a) Artist's oil paints containing barium, cadmium, or lead: use cautiously and carefully; wash hands thoroughly afterward. (b) House paints, including latex paints, containing lead or mercury (a preservative): avoid ingestion and wash carefully afterward. (c) Spray paints (the propellants are toxic): spray in a well-ventilated area.
- Cats encountered outside, other people's cats, cat litter boxes. Wild animals and birds.
- Hard drugs of any kind.

24

Enjoy!

- Good food.
- Sex.
- A sip of champagne.
- Local travel.
- Another tax deduction.
- An extra hour of sleep.
- Spreading the news.

Wrap-up

You are now over two weeks late and one month into your pregnancy. You are doubtless excited and may very well have had a positive pregnancy test by this time and know the show is definitely on the road. Your breasts are probably tender; you may be tired, have some nausea and frequency of urination, and an occasional spot of the blues (you may have some of these symptoms, all of them, or none of them). You may think that the glorious flower of motherhood, if such exists, is blooming next door because it isn't blooming with you. Nothing tastes good, nothing smells good, nothing *is* good. If this is pregnancy, you have been reading the wrong book!

If you have these problems, remember that this is all transient and will disappear later on. Besides, you may be gloriously happy. So let's get on with the show—after a little history lesson. . . .

A Primer in Obstetrical History

The history of mankind and of civilization is the history of obstetrics. As ancient tribes and cultures became structured and well ordered, so did the care of pregnant and laboring women become more special, more purposeful, and more intricate. To

25

see this unfold, it is best to divide our short history into three stages: the primitive or natural, the religious, and, finally, the scientific epoch.

Primitive or Natural Obstetrics

In this stage of human history there was an absolute lack of anatomical and physiological knowledge and, of course, no reproductive knowledge whatsoever. It is reasonable to say that the only thing figured out was the inevitable consequence of intercourse, and even that connection was not always made! No matter—what was done for the pregnant woman was what had to be done in the course of events that could not be arrested. Treatment was characterized by the simplest and crudest external manipulations, all designed to assist the natural forward motion of a child being delivered. Believe it or not, such practices continue to exist in some remote societies to this present day.

In a normal labor and delivery, certain things had to be accomplished. Instinctively women assumed a variety of positions while laboring, all to facilitate the use of bearing-down muscles to propel the infant forward. After delivery the placenta was allowed to come away spontaneously, and if it didn't, vigorous external stimulation was applied. The umbilical cord had to be severed in some fashion, the infant washed and swaddled, and the mother washed or bathed to complete the natural process. That was about it, and anybody could help.

Only a head-first delivery could be managed. Breeches and other abnormal presentations had to be converted by beating, shaking, rolling, kneading, and terrifying the laboring mother in hopes of changing the baby's position. If this failed the infant was destroyed, since it was believed to be the responsible party. Most often, sadly, the mother went with it.

The cord was severed sometime after the placenta came out. Sectioning of the cord usually took place some distance from the child's abdomen, and it was accomplished by a grinding or chewing technique. Very seldom was a sharp instrument used, because that increased the blood loss. Sometimes the cord was tied on itself; sometimes it was burned; and sometimes nothing was done to it at all.

Abortion was used for population control and was generally achieved by external beating upon—you guessed it—the mother's lower abdomen. No particular persons were assigned to "care" for laboring women, and so generally they were left in the hands of friends and relatives who had experienced labor and survived.

In more advanced but still primitive societies, some women did indeed take on the role of midwives, and it is fair to say that their "patients" did worse than when labor and delivery were managed by intuition alone. For instance, one claque of midwives in a very early Arabian setting felt the afterbirth should be left in and so avoided its expulsion if at all possible. This resulted in horrid internal putrefaction, as you might imagine. Again, another group of primitive midwives in early Chinese society felt that the placenta had to come *immediately* after the baby and, by struggling to achieve this, often turned the uterus inside out. This situation was followed very quickly by death. These times certainly favored survival of the fittest—and not even all of them! As an old cigarette ad used to say, "Nature in the raw is seldom mild!"

The Religious Epoch

We are supplied with ample evidence, in the history of the Egyptians, Indians, Greeks, and some other European cultures, of the obstetrical events of this epoch. Medical sciences sprang from the temples, as people turned to religion to drive away the evil spirits they believed caused all problems in childbearing and most other medical ills. Although labor continued to be in the hands of midwives, aid was sought from the priesthood in all difficult cases, so that they might provide divine intervention.

Thus, as time went on, priests not only did whatever that was, they further rendered effective labor assistance themselves and eventually not only performed surgical obstetrics but taught it to others. Moreover, they began to acquire a certain knowledge of anatomy and medicine and, yes, even psychological support for laboring women. They performed destructive operations on dead infants to remove them from the birth passage, and they performed cesarean sections on dead mothers to try and preserve a living child. As we approach the Dark Ages and the downfall of this epoch, we see that the Romans had goddesses for normal positions in labor and abnormal positions, for infants, for nursing, for growth and development of the fetus, and innumerable other events. Even Mena, the goddess of the monthly flow (and thus menstruation) was worshipped (and probably still is!). In the Dark Ages that followed, all obstetrical management fell back into the hands of casual midwives, and so laboring women suffered very greatly indeed. The class of women undertaking this profession was the very lowest. During the Middle Ages, after the downfall of Rome and from the sixth to the sixteenth century, darkness prevailed. Science and art were both dissipated by storms and strife and by the incursions of barbarian hordes from the east. Isolated efforts to preserve knowledge and science were crushed by the power of these tyrants, and such knowledge as survived had to be zealously guarded by the clergy within their cloistered walls. The masses were kept in the darkest ignorance and the teachings of able men were lost, laid aside, or replaced by ridiculous fetishes and practices. This was the most unfortunate period in the history of obstetrics and all of civilization.

The Scientific Period

This epoch began in the sixteenth century and continued fitfully to the present. It began with the demonstration of pelvic anatomy and with the development of some manual methods for internally or externally turning a baby that happened to be in an abnormal position. Physicians armed with newer knowledge began to find themselves invited into the birthing chamber in order to help in difficult cases. Probably the most important single step in this regard and really the true beginning of scientific obstetrics was the development of an obstetric forcep by Dr. William Chamberlayne. Physicians now had a powerful instrument to bring to the birth room, which only they could use and which could deliver children previously destined for death along with their mothers. Thus, physicians' entry into the birth chamber was guaranteed and more and more was learned about labor, pelvic anatomy, and complicated obstetrics. From that point forward the development of operative obstetrics was simply a matter of time.

That time happened to be several centuries, but progress was regular and relentless. Hastened by discoveries in other scientific fields and the development of aseptic techniques, surgical techniques, pain relief, blood transfusion, and antibiotics, we are brought into the present. It is easy to say we have reached a stage of near-perfection in the management of the laboring patient today. However, to prevent such smugness from creeping into our thoughts, one only has to read the history of obstetrics and indeed all of science to become properly humble. History and the knowledge of it serves as a great moderator of undeserved pride. One hundred years ago a famous obstetrician named Fleetwood Churchill, writing in his equally famous book, concluded that insofar as obstetrics are concerned, we had gone about as far as we could go!

Fascinating Facts

▷ The first doctor trying to get into a delivery chamber to learn more about the process dressed himself in women's clothes. He was discovered and burned to death. (His name was Von Wert, and the date was 1522.)

▷ The first doctor to prove that childbirth fever was contagious lost his hospital appointment in Vienna, was ridiculed out of his practice by his colleagues, and committed suicide. (His name: Semmelweiss; the date: 1847.)

▷ The first doctor to teach obstetrics to other doctors in America was hounded into obscurity. (His name: James P. White; the date: 1880; in Buffalo, NY.)

   . . . A little learning is a dangerous thing.

▷ Normally functioning microwave ranges, color TVs, and airport X-ray machines pose no threat during pregnancy.

DIARY

My First Month

Last period _____

Symptoms _____

_____

_____

Bleeding _____

Illness _____

_____

_____

Medications _____

_____

_____

What's going on in the world _____

_____

_____

What's going on in my life _____

_____

_____

_____

My thoughts and feelings _____

_____

_____

_____

Doctor's appointment _____

_____

Questions To Ask

_____

_____

_____

_____

_____

_____

_____

_____

_____

_____

_____

_____

_____

_____

_____

_____

_____

_____

_____

_____

_____

_____

_____

_____

CHAPTER TWO

MY SECOND
LUNAR MONTH

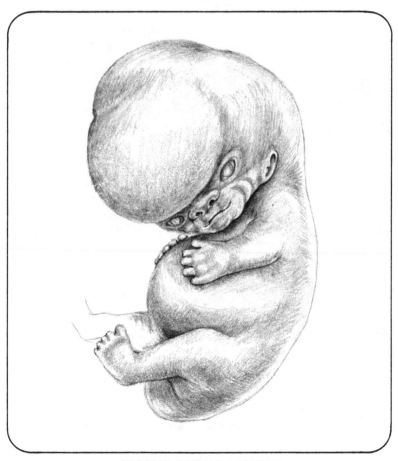

SECOND LUNAR MONTH

Having now missed your second period and having suffered one or more of the monumental initial complaints that no one else believes, you are convinced of what is going on and feel that it is time to convince the world, your doctor, and your husband of the same thing. This is about the same time that most expectant mothers call an obstetrician for their first appointment—and rightly so, because prior to this time it is usually difficult to determine for sure, without special tests, if pregnancy exists. Of course, there are exceptions to this rule, and if any of the following abnormal conditions exists, you should consult your doctor immediately:

a history of repeated miscarriages
a history of ectopic pregnancy
severe lower abdominal cramping
vaginal bleeding
severe persistent nausea or vomiting

No matter which stage of your pregnancy you feel that you are in, these conditions require immediate consultation with your doctor.

First Visit to Your Doctor

The first time you visit your obstetrician, a typical series of events will most likely occur.

Your medical history will be taken. Sometimes this history is very detailed and you will fill in a form yourself. It can contain more than one hundred questions related to your present health, past health, any previous surgery or serious illnesses you have had, any medications you are taking, family history, genetic history, even your emotional attitude toward the pregnancy. Although some questions may seem unusually detailed, they are of significant value, and your doctor must know as much as possible about your past in order to manage your pregnancy properly.

You will have a physical examination. The regular, routine physical exam includes evaluation of your whole body as well as a detailed pelvic exam. If your history reveals any significant physical or anatomical problems, special attention is given to those areas at this time. The pelvic examination determines, insofar as is possible, the presence of pregnancy, its location and duration, and whether there are any accompanying pelvic diseases or disorders, and gives an assessment of your bony pelvic structure.

Blood tests will be given and laboratory work will be done. Blood tests are taken to determine:

- your hemoglobin level and other routine blood counts
- your blood type and Rh factor
- the presence of any circulating immune antibodies in your system that might affect pregnancy
- your immunity to German measles (rubella) and toxoplasmosis (cat fever)

Further laboratory work at this time usually includes a urinalysis and a Papanicolaou smear, for routine detection of cervical

35

cancer. Note, though, that newer blood tests and procedures are commonly and constantly being added to the list of determinations made both at the initial and subsequent visits.

After the examination you and the doctor will have a consultation in which you will be given detailed advice or a book containing such advice. Necessary medications are ordered, questions are answered, the fee is established and explained, and arrangements are made for subsequent appointments.

After all this you may feel by the time you leave the doctor's office that you have forgotten your due date, your own and your doctor's names, and whether or not you put all your clothes back on! When you settle down, be sure to record your doctor's regular office phone number and emergency number in the page provided at the beginning of this book.

Subsequent Visits

If your pregnancy is quite normal, your return visits start out at monthly intervals and become progressively more frequent as time goes on. Such meetings give the doctor ample opportunity to follow your progress and for you and your doctor(s) to develop a feeling of mutual trust and confidence. Each time you return you will be weighed (the moment of truth), your blood pressure will be taken, a urinalysis will be performed, and an abdominal examination done to determine growth, development, and activity of the fetus. Sometimes certain measurements are taken as your pregnancy rises in the abdomen to correlate growth and development. The doctor either listens with a stethoscope or puts an ultrasound monitor on your abdomen, generally beginning after the twelfth week, so one or both of you can hear the developing child's heartbeat. Further special procedures may be done during your pregnancy as it progresses, particularly if there are certain complications. Just as an example, see the section on alpha fetoprotein (AFP) (p. 280) or refer to the discussion of the Rh factor on page 179.

While you are being examined, you should tell the doctor of any special problems you may have so that they may be investigated on the spot. (Remember to make note of them in the diary sections of this book.) Under normal circumstances internal examinations are not performed in the early visits, although you will probably have them toward the end of your pregnancy to reevaluate your pelvic measurements, the position of your baby, and the status of your cervix, and to determine how close you may come to your expected date of confinement. These vaginal examinations are quite safe, but since the vagina and cervix are very vascular, you may spot one or two times during the next twenty-four hours. Not to worry.

One word of caution: Although the temptation is strong, don't stop eating twenty-four hours before your regular confrontation with the scales. Doctors know from years and years of frustrating experience just how much mothers tend to shovel in. Cutting down one day before your examination won't change things very much, except that you will be weak—so weak you won't be able to stand "discussions" about weight if your doctor initiates any. Remember, you can't have your shape and eat it too. The best way to head off a lecture, by the way, is to get in there first and *lead with your list* of prepared questions!

Digestion

Morning Sickness

Most often morning sickness is a problem confined to the first three months of pregnancy. You have a fifty-fifty chance of being so affected, and even if you are, you may not be bothered very much, particularly if you follow the advice coming up. A rare few women may continue to be nauseated throughout their pregnancy, but if nausea does persist, something else is usually amiss and the doctor will find it. No one has any idea why nausea and vomiting are visitors in early pregnancy. But it is not imaginary; it is real.

If you can just hang in there you will feel better as the day goes on, since usually the nausea is a morning affair that wears off as the day progresses. But not always. You actually can be bothered by it all day and night or anytime in between, though such a degree of stomach upset is rare. (There are those who believe that this particular obstetrical problem does not exist at all or, if it does, that it is all in the mind. The nonbelievers are usually the people who have never had it—like his old girlfriend.)

Treatment of Morning Nausea

- Absolutely avoid fried, fatty, or greasy foods; highly seasoned foods (Mexican and Italian dishes, barbecue, sausage, luncheon meat, ham, etc.); and rich foods (pastries, pies, cakes, etc.).
- Concentrate on bland foods. A bland diet is outlined on pages 76–79.
- Eat frequently. Avoid big meals, and divide your daily rations into multiple small feedings that you take every hour or two insofar as possible. Try to leave food at your bedside so that if you get up at night you can nibble on a little something— like crackers, a plain cookie, or a piece of fruit. Always try to eat before you get up in the morning and before you go to bed at night; not much, but some. If you work, carry crackers, cookies, quartered sandwiches, fruit, celery sticks, carrot sticks to work. If you eat out, avoid large meals and fast-food restaurants—at this time in your life, fast foods mean fast down and fast up.
- Avoid preparations for the control of nausea and vomiting. Even though the safety margin is great, it is unwise to use any such medicines during early pregnancy. Vitamin B_6 (100 milligrams per tablet), which is not a medicine, is often used instead. It is apparently effective and quite safe. The rare cases of severe vomiting that are accompanied by dehydration,

resulting in weight loss and collapse, may require powerful medication. The risks versus the benefits of this plan must be weighed closely by you and your doctor.

- Consider taking a short leave of absence if your work requires a great deal of concentration or manual skills and if your nausea is severe. You will soon be feeling better and will want to continue your work. If, on the other hand, you have a job with a flexible work pattern, try to keep going. This is important advice at a time when you could stay home and feel very sorry for yourself, which is never good medicine.
- Be aware that some very, very few individuals become sick enough from constant vomiting to necessitate a trip to the hospital. This is particularly important if there has been enough loss of fluid to produce dehydration and to disturb the electrolyte balance in the system. Hospital treatment requires intravenous replacement of fluids, food, and electrolytes, and sometimes the use of certain drugs, as noted. Again, you and your doctor will discuss the benefit-risk ratio. Generally, the risk is severe enough that something must be done.
- Report any blood you observe in vomitus to your doctor. Very occasionally persistent vomiting produces a little blood, generally because the stomach lining is irritated. It is usually not harmful or dangerous but should be reported.

Unusual Food Cravings

Why you should suddenly crave kumquats in the middle of the night and in the dead of winter is hard to understand, but unusual food cravings are common in early pregnancy. You may give in to these desires unless they include foods that will increase your tendency to nausea or unless you crave a substance (and this is very rare) that is not a food. Strangely enough, some women experience cravings (called pica) for chalk, clay, coal, cloth, cork, turpentine, and petroleum jelly, among other things. These substances are no worse than some food offered today, but don't do it!

Mouth Watering

Sometimes an increase in the flow of saliva (ptyalism) is noted for the first few months. Again, the cause of this minor condition is unknown. There are no treatments that alter it, so that leaves us with two solutions: Either swallow it or spit it away. Neither solution is entirely agreeable—but what else can you offer?

Breasts

Though many in the wet T-shirt cult would deny it, the breasts' first reason for being is to suckle the newborn. Thus, very early in pregnancy, stimulated by fertilization, the breasts become congested and tender. Though you may have noticed in the past that your breasts were uncomfortable just before menstruation, the fullness and discomfort that occur in early pregnancy are usually somewhat greater. All of a sudden, it is distressing for you to jog, ride in a jeep, play tennis, take a shower, sleep on your stomach, make love, make haste, or do anything that moves your body faster or higher or lower or quicker than your breasts.

Your breasts will be more comfortable when supported with a well-fitting bra, but should never be bound in any way. You may even find it a relief to wear your bra while you are sleeping. If you belong to the generation that does not believe in bras, peace be with you and your breasts. Fifty percent of you will become believers in bras; the other 50 percent will become very ill tempered.

The breasts begin to grow in early pregnancy, more rapidly during the first few months and then continuing thereafter at a much slower rate. You may require a larger cup as pregnancy advances. Very rapid breast growth may be accompanied by stretch marks (striae) in the skin. Striae may be minimized somewhat by using breast support, avoiding excessive weight gain, and massaging your breasts each night with lanolin-based skin cream. I'll bet you can enlist some help here!

Sometime during pregnancy—it may be early or it may be late—a clear secretion may be noted coming from your nipples. This is colostrum, the forerunner of true milk. Milk does not appear until after delivery. The secretion of colostrum may increase during lovemaking. No problem. Finally, alas, as a result of all the pregnancy changes, your breast size may increase or decrease significantly and forever, and what was a 36 regular may end up a 36 long!

Bladder

Position means a lot in life, and it is the unfortunate position of your bladder to lie against your uterus. During pregnancy, uterine congestion puts pressure on its watery neighbor, which in turn puts pressure on you. Very early in your pregnancy you may find that a good deal of your life is spent going to and coming from your home decompression chamber. This reduced bladder capacity is somewhat overcome in the middle months of pregnancy, but as the baby's head settles down into the pelvis toward full term, your bladder once again fills at shorter intervals. Like a car with a small gas tank, your excursions are limited.

In women, the bladder is connected to the outside world by a very short tube called the urethra. When the urethra is not being used, it is kept closed by a series of muscles that you learned, long ago, to control voluntarily, and that you, if you ever want to get out of changing diapers, are shortly going to be teaching that individual in your tummy to control. As pregnancy advances, a good deal of pressure is put on the urethra, and sometimes voluntary muscular control of urination is lost, particularly when you sneeze, lift things, cough, giggle, or shout commands. This "incontinence" tends to disappear after delivery.

Infections

For a number of reasons, the bladder and the kidneys can easily become infected during pregnancy. The symptoms of lower urinary tract infection (cystitis or bladder infection) include frequent and painful urination, with a feeling of incomplete bladder emptying. Occasionally there may even be blood present and visible in the urine. On the other hand, an upper urinary tract infection (pyelitis or kidney infection) produces many of the symptoms of a lower tract infection plus chills, fever, pain high in the back on one or both sides, and feelings of acute illness. It is quite possible to have cystitis without pyelitis. You should report any of these abnormal symptoms immediately.

Drinking plenty of fluids during pregnancy will help prevent the urine from becoming too concentrated. So drink anything that isn't intoxicating, habit-forming, or polluted. Recurrent kidney infections can have an important effect upon the pregnancy and need a thorough evaluation and close monitoring.

Hospital Bladder

Various bladder problems may develop following delivery. But these will be dealt with in chapter 10.

Weariness, Fainting, and Headaches

It's July. You are downtown shopping for your husband's birthday present. Why he wants leather briefs with suede strips, God only knows, but you're doing your best—though it's hot and sticky and crowded, and the elevators are stuffed with humanity. All of a sudden a wave of nausea comes over you, the world goes black, and you collapse.

Or it's Monday morning and you're late for work—work that happens to take place on the eightieth floor of a glass tower somewhere downtown. The bus was bad enough, but now you are in a hot, stuffy elevator, you should have had breakfast, and the guy crowding you closest should not have had breakfast— or his morning cigar. At about the sixty-third-and-a-half floor you fall out, but there is nowhere to fall so nobody notices till the eightieth floor. The door opens and you fall out—for real!

Because your blood pressure is low and unstable during early pregnancy, incidents such as these are quite common. You faint because, quite literally, your brain is not getting enough blood and, therefore, not enough oxygen. The instability of your blood pressure produces other common symptoms at this time, such as weariness, dizzy spells, and, in some cases, constant dull headaches. Weariness or tiredness is probably the most common of all these complaints. If you work away from home, it is all you can do to struggle home before collapsing. If housework is your lot, you are likely to let a layer of dust settle over the house while you hibernate on the sofa.

It is important to remember that dizziness and the tendency to faint are most likely to occur when you first get up, especially if you get up too quickly, if you stand or sit too long in one position, or if you are someplace that is warm and overcrowded and you begin to feel boxed in. Try to avoid these situations. You have to get up and get going sometime, but be careful how and where you do it.

Headaches, if they occur, are usually dull and throbbing and are more likely to be constant during the day but will disappear at night—and disappear completely before midpregnancy. Don't take any medication for these headaches without consultation.

It may be tempting to quit work when you feel so tired, particularly if nausea and headaches also accompany your blood pressure instability, but you really ought to try to continue working, because these symptoms soon disappear.

Your social activities should be curtailed when they are not enjoyable or when they keep you on your feet too long. It is important for your husband to understand at this time that you feel the way you do and that it is temporary and one reason why the vows of holy matrimony include the phrase "in sickness and in health."

Prone Pressure Syndrome

Though this condition generally occurs later in pregnancy, it will be discussed here because it has to do with blood pressure instability. When your unborn babe is bigger and you lie flat on your back, the pressure against the major blood vessels and nerves running along your backbone produces a sudden and dramatic drop in blood pressure. This prone pressure syndrome is more likely to occur when you are lying down somewhere that's rather confining and you have to be still. Thus, a common place for this condition to present itself is in your doctor's office, while you wait on your back in the examining room for your doctor to get his or her act together and come in and see you. You suddenly begin to feel hot, sticky, clammy, uncomfortable, ready to faint, and generally very unhappy with your environment. If this occurs, turn immediately onto either side, but preferably onto your left side, since in this way more pressure is taken off the major blood vessels. The symptoms will disappear very quickly. The most important thing to remember is: Do not, under any circumstances, try to get up until you have been on one side or the other long enough to feel perfectly secure.

Emotions in Pregnancy

It's midnight and you have slept—if you want to call it that—for two hours. Now you're wide awake. After going to the bathroom, you turn on the Late Late Show—*Casablanca*, starring Humphrey Bogart and Ingrid Bergman. You look over at your husband, snoring happily, with his foot between you and Bogart's ear. He never needs to get up to go to the john (your husband, not Bogie). He needs his adenoids out, though! You wonder how much that would cost. And now, damn it, Ingrid is going to make the same stupid mistake that she has made the last fifty times you have seen the picture. She is going to get on the plane with that Dutchman!

While your mind is running on like this, all of a sudden, for no apparent reason, you begin to cry, to weep, and to wail. The snoring stops. Husband wakes up. Bedlam. "What's wrong? What have I done? Call the doctor. Get something to eat. Go to the bathroom. Watch TV. Do anything, but stop crying."

And so is ushered in a new and slightly disturbing companion of early pregnancy, "the blues."

Women (liberated or not) are not likely to escape episodes of emotional storms during pregnancy. Most of these storms consist of depressive interludes that come and go, usually in the early months and usually without any apparent cause. So when you have the blues and dissolve into tears and can't understand why, don't worry—and don't try to figure it out. It soon passes. Most important, be sure your husband understands that he is not the cause and that all will soon be well. Otherwise he may worry himself into a depression, and that will only make yours worse.

Medication is not necessary to control this minor depression or any of the other emotional reactions that occur during pregnancy. Generally, though, a serious preexisting emotional problem that requires regular medication must be individually dealt with by all those involved. Medication, particularly in the early months, is, as you know, best avoided. On the other hand, understanding and tolerance by all who are involved—or think they are involved—is most important. This includes sideline coaches, family prophets, and neighborhood gurus!

As pregnancy draws toward its climax, it is not unnatural for you to become somewhat apprehensive about the outcome for yourself and your baby. You may fear that the baby will be disfigured or deformed or, worst of all, will not survive. Even though you attend preparation-for-childbirth classes, you may still be apprehensive about the outcome of your labor and delivery. Further, you may fear that your relationship with your husband is jeopardized, and on and on.

You would be a most unusual person if you did not entertain these fears occasionally and even have some nightmares about them. Moreover, physical discomfort and insomnia, which occur at this time, plus any underlying problems at home, tend to add to your anxieties. Discussion of the problems with your doctor may help. Prenatal courses, too, help relieve your mind about many of the tales you may have heard or any misunderstandings you may have concerning pregnancy, labor, and delivery. Avoiding the advice and stories of well-meaning but misguided friends and relatives is probably the most important thing you can do.

You are probably aware that very shortly after delivery, "baby blues" may occur. This emotional problem generally begins the second or third day after the baby is born and is characterized by depression, crying spells, a feeling of inadequacy, and certain fears. This depression, like that of early pregnancy, is common and *temporary* in the vast majority of pregnancies. Usually it disappears just as promptly as it appeared. It will be mentioned again in the last chapter.

The most important thing you and your husband can do to promote an emotionally healthy pregnancy is to work out, insofar as you can, any tension that exists in your household. As a matter of fact, this is important not only during pregnancy but for all your married life. Problems that exist between the two of you must be brought into the open and discussed, even argued and fought over, so long as the ground rules are understood and you are working toward the resolution of a problem, a conflict, or a tension on a one-to-one basis. The development of a communication barrier between husband and wife is the death knell of their marriage. Your husband is a shareholder, not a perpetrator. You are a shareholder, not a carrier. Don't divide while you are multiplying.

Personal Hygiene

Unless you have some pretty unusual health habits, there is little to be altered in your personal hygiene during a normal pregnancy. If you have a particular complication that may interfere with ordinary hygienic routines, your doctor will give you specific instructions about what you can and cannot do. Remember, because of the changes in your body size and secretions, it is slightly more difficult to remain fastidious while you are pregnant. It is, however, important that you make every effort to do so.

Bathing and Showers

You may bathe and shower as frequently as you wish, and you may continue bathing as long as you are able to ease your body into the tub. Pregnant women have traditionally been advised to discontinue tub bathing six weeks prior to their date of delivery. No one knows why they were told this; and many of them, as you can imagine, were pretty gamy by the time labor started. The only real risk involved is getting into and out of the tub, and since you are not very agile in the last few months, be careful, but do not stop bathing.

You may take stall showers whenever you wish, but because of mechanical considerations, showering in a tub is dangerous, particularly in late pregnancy. As your balance becomes increasingly less secure, the slippery tub is much more difficult to negotiate. Thus showering in a tub should be avoided if at all possible. If you have no alternative, be sure to use a suction mat on the tub floor and to have something firm to grasp, instead of yourself, while getting in and out.

After bathing or showering, it is a good idea to lubricate your body with a skin cream containing lanolin. This is particularly true in cold, dry climates or if you have problems with dry skin anyway. Pay particular attention to your abdomen and breasts, since these areas are where the lines of pregnancy (striae) are most likely to be formed. Such lines can be minimized by keeping your skin well lubricated.

Hot Tubs

This form of communal or semicommunal bathing is becoming popular, and so spending prolonged periods of time in a hot tub doing whatever—or nothing—is not uncommon. There is *very strong evidence* that this is not a good game to play during pregnancy, because significant elevations of body temperature, as such bathings accomplish, can have harmful fetal effects. Moreover, most private hot tubs are not very sanitary, and they can become a collection point for bacteria that can be harmful and unpleasant to you. Public spa facilities are required to keep the water in their saunas and tubs relatively sterile. However, again, recent evidence shows that plastic surfaces such as the benches used in these areas can culture positively for viruses, including the herpes virus. So—be careful.

If you avoid the risks, then, bubble, oil, mud, sauna, Turkish, Swedish, Japanese, mineral, milk, and champagne baths are all acceptable. Just be sure to take good care of yourself and anoint yourself with oil and keep clean and, as indicated, keep cool— no prolonged heat exposure.

Your Hair

In addition to shampooing, you may continue to tease, twist, tip, rat, set, curl, blow-dry, and otherwise mutilate your hair, with this important limitation: Avoid any dyes during pregnancy or, for that matter, any chemicals on your hair.

It is of value to note here that some changes that occur in hair during pregnancy may or may not involve your own locks. Some women have magnificent curly hair. This may be a blessing, depending upon current hairstyles. Nevertheless, pregnancy sometimes straightens the curl, temporarily or permanently, and there is nothing you can do about it. Further, your hair may become dryer, requiring you to change your shampooing habits. Finally, sometime after you deliver—usually during the second to fourth months—you may notice a sudden loss of scalp hair. This hair regrows, and the scalp hair density begins to appear normal in about six months, though for some women regrowth may take much longer, tempting them to resort to wigs—and why not? *Very rarely* it will not regrow at all and your hair will remain permanently somewhat thinner. Remembering this when you go home after delivery, you should avoid trauma to your hair for the first six months. Thus postpone, if you can, the use of rollers, pincurls, permanent-wave solutions, teasing, straightening, and other abusive hair treatment. You should use a natural-bristle hairbrush and keep vigorous hairbrushing to a minimum. Shampoo as often as necessary.

Douching

During pregnancy, normal vaginal secretions often increase because of the marked local congestion. Such secretions are generally white and should not be offensive or cause any irritation or itching. It is important to note, though, that certain vaginal infections are common during pregnancy and produce

49

a discharge that is either offensive or irritating or both (see pp. 104–110).

Some physicians feel it is not safe to douche during pregnancy, but many others agree that under the proper circumstances, no harm will occur. If you wish to continue to douche and your doctor doesn't restrict it, remember the following rules.

In the event of any bleeding or discomfort, discontinue douching at once. Do not douche in the last month of your pregnancy, because at that time the baby sits low in the pelvis and douching may be dangerous and certainly uncomfortable.

Use bag-and-flow gravity equipment. The bag is supported above the body and allows irrigating liquid to flow into the vagina by gravity alone. At no time during pregnancy should syringe-type douching equipment be employed. Unless otherwise instructed, use clear water for douching or add a tablespoon of vinegar to a quart of water. No other douching materials should be used in the vagina unless prescribed by your physician.

Exercises and Athletics

Exercise. If you have a brace of little ones at home underfoot, you had better skip this section: You get sufficient exercise, though perhaps not the kind you want—or need.

There is much discussion among physicians (there always is—about everything) regarding whether special exercises are necessary to help women enhance the success of their pregnancy. After all, they go on, women were built for the job, and it would appear that most normally active young women should be able to deliver without extra physical preparation. However, there is ample evidence that most American women do not get sufficient active exercise to be well prepared for childbirth. This deficiency may gradually be changing as greater emphasis is being put on personal health and exercise programs. It is certainly clear that labor is much simpler physically and emo-

50

tionally among those who have had some education and special exercise preparation in their prenatal planning.

The most commonly advocated form of exercise in pregnancy is walking. Here, again, women who work and those who lead an active life usually get sufficient walking activity during the day without resorting to extra excursions. Nevertheless, walking is good and helpful; a moderate but not excessive form of exercise. Jogging is also of great value, not only for its exercise potential but also for keeping the cardiovascular system well toned and tuned.

The standard sitting-up exercises are also perfectly acceptable during normal pregnancy. If you wish to work out at the corner health and fitness salon, most of the gadgets they provide are compatible with pregnancy. The possible exception might be vibrator belts and roller machines.

There are special books available nowadays detailing aerobic and other exercises specifically tailored to pregnant women. And in the main, all of them are helpful, and all of their programs may be followed in a healthy pregnancy upon which your physician has placed no special restrictions.

Finally, if you are attending a prepared childbirth class now or have in a previous pregnancy, you will have been given special exercises that will be of value to you during labor and delivery.

Sports

You may participate in most of the usual sport activities, provided you do not have a history of repeated miscarriage or of premature labor. Under such circumstances, your doctor will give you special instructions about your activities.

The philosophy behind allowing you to continue sports— even some physically demanding ones—is that you are mature enough to accept certain risks involved in return for the many benefits that result. Some danger exists in all athletic endeavors whether or not you are pregnant, and you are aware of this fact when you decide that you are going to ride, or jump, or dive, or ski, or do anything physical. The difference now is that you are sharing the risks with another human being—your baby. Generally, the exercise and fulfillment obtained in such physical endeavors outweigh the danger involved. And besides, there are risks in just getting up in the morning!

We note, for example, a reported case of a pregnant woman who was struck very hard in the abdomen with a softball. She miscarried. It is most likely that the forceful blow to her abdomen produced the miscarriage. We have also seen that even light blows to the abdomen from a steering wheel can produce a miscarriage. So there are chances that we must be prepared to accept if we are not going to shut ourselves away from all activity. Even then, the roof may cave in!

Now, you were cautioned earlier to avoid violent athletic physical activity at all costs. This is the area of competitive physical activity that strains muscles to the end point of tolerance, such as mountain climbing, judo, tournament tennis, swimming, and running. Exertions of this kind can be dangerous to your pregnancy because they drain blood away from central vital organs, including the uterus, and thereby siphon oxygen from your baby. Avoid sports that produce sudden changes in oxygen transference—this includes scuba diving, unpressurized flying, and snow skiing—till you adjust to the altitude change (it takes about 48 hours).

A recent broad assessment of female participation in athletics made by a knowledgeable group of physicians concluded that the physiological and social benefits to be gained through the physical activity of recreational sports and competition far outweigh any risks. In many cases, they add, physical activity improved the distinctive biological functions of the female. Whatever that means.

Unfortunately, you may, under normal circumstances, continue to do housework and yard work with little fear of producing anything other than grubby nails, an aching back, or hay fever.

Working

Many women who work become pregnant, and vice versa. Pregnant women entered the labor force in significant numbers during World War II, and the trend has continued. Thus, since over 60 percent of married women are now employed, the relationship between work and pregnancy comes up very often. Of interest, let's note that the armed services have now designed maternity uniforms! Next it will be space suits.

The questions that come up, of course are:

Can I continue to work?
How long can I continue to work?
What could make a temporary leave necessary?
What types of work are dangerous for pregnant women?
When should I return to work?

The answers to these questions involve three factors:

the expectant mother's health
the type of work
company policy

Ordinarily, a healthy pregnant woman may continue to work as long as she continues being healthy, in a reasonable environment, doing work that does not involve agility in late pregnancy. It is probably better to continue to work than to suffer boredom and "food-in-mouth" disease at home. The distress of working is considerably less than the stress of staying home.

What pregnant women should not work? Pregnant women with any of the following conditions probably should not work:

• repeated premature labor and repeated abortions

- moderately severe or severe heart disease
- blood diseases producing marked anemia, such as sickle cell anemia or thalassemia
- hypertension
- certain categories of diabetes
- certain other disabilities (e.g., women who are chronic asthmatics or who have severe back problems)

The following types of employment are probably best avoided by pregnant women:

- radiology or any work with radiation, unless rigorously monitored
- work involving exposure to anesthetic gases
- veterinary medicine or work in pet shops
- teaching, under some circumstances, particularly if the expectant mother is not immunized to German measles (rubella), or if there are posture problems, such as backaches, varicose veins, etc.
- work in hospitals, oral surgeons' offices, dialysis units, and other areas where the risk of hepatitis is high
- work in factories producing or using chemical substances known to affect pregnancy (see following list)

The following chemicals have known harmful effects on pregnancy, and work involving these agents should be avoided:

- heavy metals, such as cadmium, lead, mercury
- organic solvents, such as benzene
- certain hydrocarbons, such as vinyl chloride, ethylene debromide, PCB, DMP, and chloroprene
- hypoxic agents, such as carbon monoxide
- anesthetic gases, such as halogenated gases
- pesticides
- estrogens, such as DES (used in cattle and poultry processing)

This list is fairly complete, but new substances are being added daily. So check with your doctor.

Company Policies

Most organizations have a policy with regard to pregnant employees, designed to protect both the organization and the mother. In the past many of these policies have been unrealistic and have discriminated against pregnant women. These restrictive policies are gradually disappearing, and those that are left are more and more being challenged in the courts. If you feel that work restrictions in your organization are unfair, you may take your employer to court, but be warned that the decision may come in time for your grandchildren's benefit. It is usual now for seniority and other benefits to continue undisturbed after pregnancy.

Leave of Absence

It is not uncommon, as we have already seen (for instance, if nausea and vomiting occur), for a short-term illness to make it wise to take a temporary leave of absence. Infectious diseases such as influenza and even the common cold are harder to combat and shake off during pregnancy than at other times. Temporary anemias may require a leave of absence while the blood count builds back. Whenever these short-term illnesses and disorders come up, it is probably wiser to take a leave of absence than to stop working completely.

Return to Work

The customary time to return to work after either a normal vaginal delivery or a cesarean section is six weeks. If there have been undue complications, such as infection, anemia, blood loss, or any other problems of the delivery and the recovery period, your physician will give you a special work return time, and most companies honor the decision.

55

These working guidelines are just that—guidelines. There are many variations, and the principles laid down here are like the perforations provided to open a box of facial tissues. It's very seldom that the true course of events exactly follows the lines laid out.

Discomfort in Early Pregnancy

There are several sorts of discomfort in the lower abdomen that are not uncommon in early pregnancy, though they are usually in no way serious.

Cramps

Slight menstrual-type cramps are apt to occur, particularly at the time you are missing a period. Your uterus questions its new passenger, which is stretching its walls, and so it cramps back ever so lightly. These pains may last a day or two but are very moderate in nature. If the cramping should become severe or be associated with any spotting whatsoever, your doctor should be called at once, as this is an abnormal sign and needs some observation.

Ligament Pain

Very commonly in the early months of pregnancy, the uterus, as it grows, turns slightly to one side or the other, but more often to the right. Such twisting produces a pulling pain, usually in the lower right side of the abdomen. You will notice it most frequently when you get up quickly or turn sharply from one side to the other, and you may feel it on both sides. This pain is present only in the early months of pregnancy and is just nagging in nature, of no real significance. Any other pain in the lower abdomen or pain that is crippling should be reported.

56

Other Pain

The existence of a corpus luteum cyst during the first few months of pregnancy may cause some pain. This cyst forms at the very spot on your ovary from which you ovulated. It creates the hormone progesterone, which normally helps support your pregnancy. But you already know that.

Fascinating Facts

▷ You can sleep in a water bed. After all, that's what your baby is sleeping in.

▷ Many mothers who are heavy smokers and can't seem to quit, even knowing the risks to their babies, will completely put away cigarettes after watching their first ultrasound procedure. Something about the little child's heartbeat or body movements turns mother on and nicotine off.

DIARY

My Second Month

Any problems _____

Illness _____

_____

Medications _____

_____

Spotting _____

Persistent nausea, etc. _____

_____

Travel _____

_____

Ultrasound—Why? _____

_____

What's going on in the world? _____

_____

What's going on in my life? _____

_____

My thoughts and feelings _____

_____

Doctor's appointment _____

Questions To Ask

CHAPTER THREE

MY THIRD
LUNAR MONTH

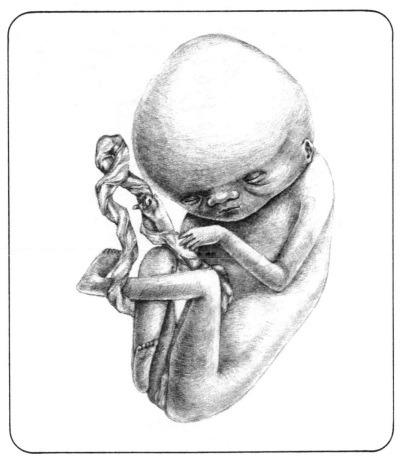

THIRD LUNAR MONTH

Your baby is fully formed now and is about as big as a large rosebud. Its heart is and has been beating. It is moving about, but you probably cannot feel any movements because it is still too small. Your uterus is the size of a large orange.

Now, nearing the point of missing your third period and entering the third lunar month of your pregnancy, you are about to pass a physiological landmark. Several changes take place. One of them concerns the hormone progesterone, which, as you know, is vitally important to the maintenance of pregnancy. Until now this hormone has been secreted almost entirely by the ovary (the corpus luteum cyst), but hereafter it will be secreted by the placenta (afterbirth). This transference of hormone manufacture does not always progress smoothly. It is at this time in pregnancy, therefore, that one type of spontaneous abortion may take place.

Spontaneous Abortions

Strictly speaking, *abortion* is a medical term that means the loss of a pregnancy before the fetus can survive. The popular term for this is *miscarriage.* The causes of spontaneous abortion are frequently multiple, very complex, and often unrecognized. It is now known that up to 80 percent of all conceptions do not result in a live birth! This is startling information, but let me hasten to point out that most of these pregnancies pass undetected and may not even cause a delay in menstruation.

Now then, the likelihood that a *recognized* pregnancy will end in spontaneous abortion is about 25 percent—one in four pregnancies is destined to end in abortion. Why is this? Well, the human reproductive process is extremely efficient in screening conceptions for normality. Thus, 97 percent of *recognized* human pregnancies with genetic defects are aborted spontaneously. Only the very few remaining go on to result in a live birth or a stillbirth of a child with chromosomal defects. Indeed, at least half of all abortions are related to genetic defects. The other causes of spontaneous abortion are:

anatomical defects in the uterus
systemic maternal disorders, such as chronic kidney and heart
    disease, diabetes, and thyroid problems
infectious diseases such as cytomegalovirus, toxoplasmosis, and
    chlamydia
hormone defects in the reproductive system
blood group incompatibility
age of mother
injury
environmental and social poisons, such as tobacco, alcohol, etc.

The commonest time for spontaneous abortion is at the eleventh to twelfth week. The next most likely is at the seventh week. Finally, about 2½ percent of women who reach the sixteenth week of pregnancy abort before the twenty-eighth week. This figure is important to remember when considering the risks involved in invasive procedures such as amniocentesis, which may be blamed for abortions that were about to happen anyway.

The symptoms of an impending abortion are vaginal bleeding and menstrual-type cramping. Promptly report to your doctor any abnormal bleeding and anything other than slight cramping at the time a period is being missed. If you have a history of repeated early abortions, your doctor will give you more intensive care and certain special instructions concerning limitation of your activity. If hormones are of value, they may be given.

When abortion is inevitable, has already begun, or is partially completed, it is most likely that you will be admitted to the hospital, where a curettement (a scraping of the uterus, popularly known as a D and C) will probably be performed.

It is very important to remember and to believe that one abortion does not necessarily predispose a person to a second. Not often do conditions exist that repeatedly produce abortion. And the patient who habitually aborts can many times have normal pregnancies after proper surgery, after hormone therapy is instituted, or after existing disorders and infections are controlled. Rh-negative women may need Rh-vaccination after an abortion. Be sure to check this with your physician.

The management of threatened abortion is becoming much simpler and the prediction of fetal survival much better, in that we are able to use, in combination, ultrasound monitoring and the beta HCG pregnancy test. Generally, if the HCG levels are doubling every day and the ultrasound shows continued evidence of fetal growth and activity, we have a healthy, stable situation. Once the tenth week is reached and fetal cardiac activity is present, growth and development are on schedule, and the beta HCG level is climbing, then the outcome of pregnancy is almost always successful. These techniques further help us in determining pregnancies that cannot and will not survive, and therefore useless therapy and increasing emotional involvement can be halted.

Hobbies

According to a recent survey, around 60 million Americans are involved in hobby crafts of some sort. Hobbies are an excellent way to relax and are a healthy form of self-expression. Few hobbies constitute a real threat to pregnancy, but many chemical compounds find their way into the hobbyist's equipment; therefore, it is important to determine if any of these may be harmful.

Since there now exist about two and a half million chemical compounds, with more being added each and every year, it is important that the relationship of hobbyists and chemicals to pregnancy, insofar as possible, be defined.

There is truth to the old saying that painting endangers a pregnant woman and her child. Insofar as oil painting is concerned, certain pigments are derivatives of lead, cadmium, barium, and other heavy metals. Although there is almost no danger of inhaling these substances while you are painting, you may accidentally ingest some of them from your fingers or they may work through the skin. Do not hold brush handles in your mouth. All pigments, particularly lead, which accumulates in the body, can be harmful to both mother and child. Even though painting may not be your hobby, you may feel called upon to paint a room or some piece of furniture during pregnancy. No matter what the calling is, avoid lead-based paint. If you paint indoors, use synthetic paint in a well-ventilated room.

Most house paints, including latex paints, contain a small amount of mercury to prevent mildew and spoilage. If this is ingested or gets to the intestines in any way (via the lungs and bloodstream, for instance), it could be converted to a type of mercury that is damaging to the fetus. Though no studies are available to indicate that the mercury in our paint is of a high enough level to cause any trouble, why take the chance? Be sure that you paint in a well-ventilated area, and keep paint off your body, making certain that none remains on you when you are through. You may even get out of painting altogether!

If your hobbies run to metal sculpture, in which there is a possibility of noxious gases accumulating, or to the construction of miniature airplanes, autos, trains, and so on, or any other conceivable activity involving fumes from glues or sprays, be sure to work in a well-ventilated area.

Barium cobalt oxide and lead are commonly used as glazes in pottery. These agents are toxic, and contact with them, particularly with the lead, should be avoided. Other materials, such as asbestos used in modeling material and sawdust as a result of carpentry work, represent a hazard to you because they can cause lung disorders. If your hobby runs to photography, please stay out of the darkroom and away from its chemicals. Another dark room has already caused you enough trouble.

Clothing

Time was, when a pregnant woman outgrew her regular clothes she retired to her home, out of public view. This is how the word *confinement* came to be related to pregnancy: She literally was confined to her home until the blessed event. There were no maternity clothes and little discussion about maternity or clothes. What mothers put on their bodies is not known to us. All we know is that they were well covered and lonely as the devil.

Today expectant mothers carry their precious burdens every-where throughout all of pregnancy, and they expect and deserve to be covered with comfortable garments. The clothing industry has met this challenge with a great variety of good-looking maternity clothes that you should begin to wear as soon as your regular clothes become uncomfortable. This time arrives differ-ently for each expectant mother and each pregnancy, depending on weight and build, how many pregnancies you have enjoyed, the size of this pregnancy, and what you put into your stomach. When your time for maternity clothes comes, don't fight it. You will be sick and tired of wearing maternity clothes before you are finished, but at least you will be sick and tired in comfort. Some other points:

• Try one of the many attractive swimsuits for pregnant women. You may continue to swim throughout a normal pregnancy.
• Wear comfortable and well-fitting shoes. Avoid high heels

and pointed toes, because they represent a very unstable underpinning. Incidentally, your foot size may increase slightly during pregnancy, and may never decrease. More good news.

- Never wear round garters to support your hose. Wear either maternity garter belts or pantyhose designed for pregnant women. If you are troubled with varicose veins during your pregnancy, fairly attractive support hose and support pantyhose can be purchased and should be used. Pregnant or not, you should wear pantyhose with a cotton crotch. Synthetic fibers trap moisture in the vulvovaginal area, resulting in odor and a tendency, which already exists in pregnancy anyway, to vaginal infections; further, the dampness makes such infections harder to cure.

- Do you have to wear a bra during pregnancy? You don't *have* to, but good judgment dictates that you get some support when you need it. Remember, colostrum may stain your bra, or if you don't choose to wear one, it will stain the next closest garment. Disposable nursing shields protect your bra or whatever.

Your Weight

Having lived through the agony and deprivation caused by nausea, many women become obsessed with the need to make up for lost time foodwise. Everything edible looks, tastes, smells, even feels good. Your passions no longer ignite for your old stablemate, furs, diamonds, Yves St. Laurent, or Elizabeth Barrett Browning's sonnets. Instead you are now turned on by fried chicken, creamed potatoes—creamed anything—ice cream, pies, cakes, rolls, cookies, doughnuts, or dough anything. You, dear one, have "food-in-mouth" disease. Soon, however, you discover that your continuing orgy is associated with a few problems. First, your scale begins to register your weight incorrectly and so does the doctor's scale—always on the high side, of course. Next thing you know, the washing machine is ruining everything you own: something in it is making all your clothes shrink so that nothing fits any part anymore. Finally, and worst of all, your family and friends don't look at you eye-to-eye while talking to you. No, they let their gaze wander all over the magnificent extent of your body!

This brings us to a head-on confrontation with cooking and corpulence during pregnancy. First of all, here are some facts to contemplate.

1. The United States ranks only fourteenth in the world in infant salvage at birth and until recently has been losing ground—unbelievable but true. One of the major contributing factors to this sad truth is the poor dietary habits of American expectant mothers. Other things are involved, but diet is extremely important. (Denmark, incidentally, is number one in the world in fetal survival.) You are what you eat. The substance of your body organs and tissues can come from no other source than the food you ingest. You cannot hope to grow a baby if you do not have the building blocks stored in your body or do not supply them in your dietary intake.

2. Adolescent mothers are more common in the United States than in any other civilized country. These adolescent pregnancies are increasing both relatively and actually. The growing youngster who becomes pregnant faces many more physiological risks than her completely developed sister, and not the least of these is the fact that she has undertaken to develop another human being before the growth of her own body is completed. This produces many nutritional hazards, and adolescent mothers lose more children at birth than any other category of pregnant women in the United States.

3. Available evidence on the nutritional status and food habits of American mothers, both pregnant and not pregnant, suggests that their dietary habits are often inadequate and

bizarre. The intake of iron, calcium, certain vitamins, and proteins is well below what it should be. Iron deficiency is very common, with not enough to meet the expectant mother's iron needs let alone those of the growing infant. The likelihood of iron-deficiency anemia in both mother and child is very great indeed. The iron supplement provided for pregnant women, even if taken according to instructions, is often inadequate to supply these demands. After that lecture, I am sure you will read and follow the pregnancy diet outline that begins on page 74.

There are three ways of gaining weight during pregnancy, and unfortunately, two of them involve eating—usually good eating. The growing infant and associated structures account for about seventeen pounds of your total weight gain. Included in this amount is the actual weight of the baby at birth, the afterbirth (placenta), the amniotic fluid, the increase in the size of your uterus and breasts, and the additional blood in your system. Over this seventeen-pound addition to your weight you have little control, but weight gain is also caused by the deposit within you of fats and fluids or both. Over these two you can exercise more control.

Provided you are not overweight when you first conceive, an increase of five to ten pounds in your *own* weight is acceptable during your pregnancy and, according to some recent evidence, may actually improve the health of your newborn child. Thus a total pregnancy weight gain in the area of 25 pounds is now considered about right. An infant's birth weight is largely established by genetic factors and by the length of time your baby is within you. But certain diseases, certain drugs (nicotine and heroin, for instance), and certain pregnancy disorders can also markedly alter newborn birth weight. Moreover, chronic malnutrition has marked effects on fetal weight as well as on fetal well-being. You already know this.

A word to the wise: If you are overweight at the beginning

of your pregnancy, you are at a disadvantage, but your doctor will probably not attempt to make you lose weight during your pregnancy. Do not, on your own, attempt any crash diets, any fad diets, or any other restrictive measures to lose weight slowly, suddenly, or in *any* amount while you are pregnant.

Recap

• Usual weight gain:
  baby, placenta, amniotic fluid, uterine and breast growth, extra blood—17 pounds
  your body growth—8 pounds
  average pregnancy gain—25 pounds
• Excessive real gain (*excludes* fluid retention) may not be harmful but is very, very hard to lose after the event.
• Do not panic if you are not gaining as much as the average allows. If you are eating well and feeling well, and your doctor says your passenger is well, then all else is most likely well.
• The rate of weight gain seems to increase as pregnancy advances; in the second half this amounts to a pound a week.
• Do not diet or try to lose weight.

Fat

Fat is deposited when the body takes in more food than it requires. This extra food is converted into fat and stored. It is unfortunate but true that all conditions are in favor of your getting and holding fat in your body during pregnancy. After you have delivered, nothing is in favor of your losing it. Though the excess fat you put on during pregnancy does not harm you or your pregnancy in any real way that we know of, it harms you if it stays with you afterward.

If you would like to understand how thirty pounds of excess fat can harm you if it stays with you, then you might try the following experiment sometime when you are not pregnant. Some morning when you get up, haul out six 5-pound bags of sugar and tie them around your waist. Carry them around with you all day, doing whatever you ordinarily do, and see how you feel by the end of the day. See how quickly you tire and get short of breath, and notice how rapidly your heart beats. Now if you are, say, thirty pounds overweight, you not only have to carry this weight around with you constantly but you first must buy it, eat it, and store it; then carry it, feed it, bathe it, warm it, cool it, dress it, get rid of its waste, and do everything else for it, day in and day out for as long as you have it. This partially explains why the life expectancy of an individual decreases proportionally to the amount of his or her extra weight.

Fluids

Gaining weight through the retention of fluid may involve danger. During pregnancy certain hormones are produced that partially blunt your kidneys' ability to excrete fluid. Fluids tend to build up in the bloodstream and spill into the body's tissues. This fluid retention is for some reason more likely to occur in warm, humid weather and when there are marked shifts in barometric pressure. You may notice that by the end of the day your legs are very swollen and uncomfortable, particularly if you stand or sit at work. Gravity has pulled the fluid toward your lower extremities. When you go to bed, the fluid redistributes itself throughout the body. It has *not* disappeared; it has just moved to its nighttime quarters. Furthermore, the wide swings that can occur in your weight, particularly in the last few months of pregnancy, are also due to sudden retention or release of body fluids.

In trying to control fluid retention, do not restrict your intake of water or other liquids. This is of no value, and in fact it is important to maintain an adequate intake of fluids throughout pregnancy. To deal with accumulated fluid in your lower extremities, it is a good idea, if you have a sitting job, to get up and move around; when you have a break period, try to lie down with your legs elevated. If you are on your feet at home a great deal, lie down whenever you have a chance, with your feet elevated.

Weight due to water retention will not stay with you or add to your permanent weight in any way. But it is sometimes a very uncomfortable and painful side effect of your pregnancy and, in my opinion, of your diet.

The role of salt in the retention of fluid is very important. In the past doctors restricted salt intake very vigorously in pregnant women because they felt it was a dangerous substance that increased the chances of developing hypertension of pregnancy. This is a disease the frequency of which, fortunately, is gradually diminishing. Also called, in the past, toxemia, preeclampsia, or poisoning of pregnancy, it has a triad of symptoms: high blood pressure, retention of fluids, and albumen in the urine. The retention of fluid in this condition is pathological and must be treated differently (see hypertension of pregnancy, page 156).

We now know that salt is not the basic culprit in pregnancy hypertension. But excessive salt intake is a great danger to all of us because it is closely related to the development of high blood pressure. Most Americans consume a great excess of sodium, mainly as salt, in their diet each day. I would recommend that you salt your food very, very lightly and avoid excessively salted food as much as you can.

Water pills (diuretics) are available to help remove excess fluid from your body. However, it is not wise to take these powerful drugs during normal pregnancy to reduce your collection of body fluid. They have many side effects that are undesirable during pregnancy—or anytime—one of them being to wash important electrolytes out of your bloodstream and your body along with the wasted water.

Calories

A calorie is a unit of energy given off by a measured amount of food as it is burned in the body. Different foods have different caloric values. A stick of celery has almost no calories, whereas an equal amount of chocolate torte covered with whipped cream provides about 900 calories. You could eat celery all day and not gain a bit, but one bite of the torte would be about half your basic daily requirement. An unfortunate fact is that foods we don't necessarily enjoy are low in caloric value, and vice versa. Any standard cookbook contains a list of caloric equivalents; you can find this section easily by looking for the pages that are not dog-eared.

Throughout the day in my office I hear excuses given by mothers-to-be as they try to slither out of their weight problems. Don't use them. Doctors have heard them all before.

Instead of excuses, you can try two other little gambits to avoid the doctor's wrath—you can try tidbits or tears. A moist eye is hard to level with, and so is a moist home-baked brownie. Besides, how can any doctor put down a gift-bearer and a bread-sharer? Try these approaches.

Your obstetrician may make no mention at all about your weight gain unless you have some abnormality in your pregnancy, such as hypertension. He or she may feel that weight control is your problem. Perhaps it is, but many doctors are distressed to watch a 120-pound beauty end up a 160-pound spread—and they know that depression will follow when, after delivery, the mother discovers how hard it is to get that weight off.

Your Daily Bread

Regular Pregnancy Diet

The perfect diet for pregnant women is yet to be discovered. Ideally, it should contain protein, vitamins, and minerals to satisfy the growing baby; fats, sweets, sugar, and salt to satisfy its ravenous mother; and melting agent X, which eats away pounds to satisfy a nagging doctor. Since nothing even close to that exists, here's what you're left with:

- **Meat, fish, poultry.** Eat these foods at least twice a day, and favor fish and poultry over red meat. All these fleshes contain animal protein. Try not to fry the fish and poultry; broil, poach, roast, or bake instead. Make a pass at liver occasionally, if you can. Meat should be lean. Hamburgers aren't lean.
- **Dairy products.** More animal protein. Have some each day.

    Eggs. Eat two eggs daily or bury them in some sort of recipe. Contrary to popular belief, eggs do not have to be fried to be eaten; they can be boiled, shirred, coddled, poached, scrambled, omeleted, or eaten raw.
    Cheese. Acceptable if digestible.
    Milk. A controversial food. If you are hooked on it, drink skim milk—and not much of it—always making sure you get adequate protein and calcium from other sources. This is in contradiction of conventional pregnancy diet instructions. You will discover why later on (see pages 200–201). Yogurt is a good substitute for milk.

- **Vegetables.** Have plenty of all kinds each day, with few limitations.

74

Corn and potatoes contain starch, which turn to sugar in your stomach on the way to becoming fat. Restrict your intake of these vegetables if you are overweight or gaining rapidly.

Green leafy vegetables are a great source of bulk and iron; eat lots of these.

- **Fruit.** Fine food. Eat all kinds, if fresh, daily. Canned fruits are generally heavily sugared, so if you are overweight you can get dietetic canned fruits at your supermarket. Don't put salt on melon. Fruits are excellent for dessert if served without ice cream, whipped cream, or any other kind of cream.
- **Rice.** Though starchy, like potatoes, rice contains protein and is excellent as a substitute.
- **Bread, pies, cakes, cookies, pastries, rolls, buns.** These are full of sugar, starch, baking soda, salt, butter, and air. Therefore, they are instant sources of energy and gas; if energy is not required, they are a great source of instant fat. Restrict their use somewhat if you are gaining excessively. Whole wheat is a better daily bread than white.
- **Prepared cereals.** Fine. But some prepared cereals are, unfortunately, mainly sugar. Read the package label. Add skim milk and just a little sugar.
- **Salads.** Great. Instead of salad dressings, try lemon juice, or oil and vinegar, or oil and red table wine. Avoid salads with onion, garlic, radish, peppers, or other irritating vegetables when you are nauseated or have heartburn.
- **Diet drinks.** Soft drinks and diet drinks that contain caffeine should probably be avoided. Otherwise they are safe. Regular soft drinks have the added disadvantage of a high sugar content, which, again, adds to your calories.

During the last half of your pregnancy, limit salt and salty foods as well as foods that contain baking soda. Various seasoning substitutes may be used and will be found on pages

82–83. Low-salt and low-sodium foods can be found in the dietetic-foods section of your supermarkets. In fact, many canned vegetables now in your supermarket are being offered salt-free. This is in response to the tremendous amount of evidence indicating the dangers of our oversalted society.

Low-calorie foods with artificial sweeteners are acceptable, when necessary.

Whiskey, beer, and wine should be consumed with great caution in pregnancy. This is mentioned over and over in other sections of this book. These substances can be exceedingly dangerous to your baby. Further and perhaps less important, if you are overweight: beer is 100 calories per average glass; whiskey, 85; a martini, 150; a glass of wine, 100. Just extra sources of fat building. On the other hand, if you have a poor appetite, one ounce of dry sherry (140 calories) taken very occasionally before a meal often stimulates hunger. Beer is helpful for nursing mothers because it increases their fluid intake pleasantly and is also somewhat relaxing, except to the bladder.

On request, your doctor will give you a safe low-calorie diet if your weight gain must be limited. Do not try to lose weight while you are pregnant unless your doctor orders it for some reason. Do not count calories unless you are overweight or gaining at an excessive rate. If weight is a problem, avoid food and drink high in calories but low in nutritional value.

For further free information on diets, request the booklet *Food, Pregnancy and Family Health* from the American College of Obstetricians and Gynecologists, 600 Maryland Avenue Southwest, Washington, D.C. 20024.

Bland Diet

A bland diet is for old millionaires, nervous executives, and expectant mothers who have nausea and vomiting or heartburn. The principles involved in this bland diet include the following:

(1) You must not add anything to your stomach that further irritates it and (2) you must not let your stomach get empty— or full.

Serve the following every day:

- **Milk.** Three or more cups, skimmed.
- **Eggs.** One or more, poached, soft- or hard-cooked, scrambled, as an omelet.
- **Meat or alternative.** Two servings daily (at least one of these should be meat, fish, poultry, or game) of beef, lean ham, veal, lamb, pork (trimmed of excess fat), fish (including shellfish), poultry, or game—broiled, baked, boiled, or creamed. Meats should be ground if they are not tender. Canned salmon or tuna in water, cottage cheese, Swiss or cheddar cheese, and smooth peanut butter are good alternatives.

  Avoid: fried eggs; fried, fatty and greasy meats; highly seasoned ham, smoked meats, wieners, bologna, luncheon meats, sausage, salt pork, corned beef; mackerel, sardines; strong-flavored cheese; chunky peanut butter; dried beans and peas.

- **Potato or alternative.** One serving of white potato or sweet potato, boiled, mashed, creamed, scalloped, or baked. Enriched rice, grits, macaroni, noodles, or spaghetti may be substituted for potato but not served at the same meal.

  Avoid: fried potato, potato chips, corn, hominy, dried beans and peas.

- **Vegetables.** Two servings or more, of which one is a dark green or deep yellow vegetable, at least every other day. Raw tender lettuce; cooked or canned tender asparagus tips, beans (only baby lima, green, yellow wax), beets, frozen black-eyed peas, carrots, eggplant, green peas, mushrooms, pumpkin, spinach, winter squash, tomato juice or puree (unseasoned).

  Avoid: fried and greasy vegetables; raw vegetables (except lettuce); broccoli; brussels sprouts; cabbage; cauliflower;

cucumbers; greens such as escarole, chicory, and dandelion; okra; onions; parsnips; radishes; rutabagas; summer
squash; tomatoes (except puree or juice); turnips; and
any others you find difficult to digest.

- **Fruits.** Two servings or more. One should be an orange or
a grapefruit or its juice. Ripe banana, avocado, or tangerine;
peeled apples, nectarines, peaches, pears, or plums; unpeeled
apricots and cherries; strained rhubarb sauce, strained stewed
dried fruits, or any fruit juices.

    Avoid: raw fruits other than those listed; cooked fruits
    with coarse fibers, skins, or seeds, such as pineapple,
    berries, figs, prunes, fruit cocktail.

- **Bread and cereal.** Four servings or more. Enriched white,
whole wheat, or light rye bread, and rolls without seeds; thin
biscuits and cornbread; plain coffeecake; plain cinnamon
rolls; rusks; Melba toast; zwieback; salt crackers; graham
crackers; cocktail crackers without seeds; any cooked cereals,
such as oatmeal, cream of wheat, cream of rice, etc.; enriched
dry cereals.

    Avoid: coarse dark breads and breads with seeds, pancakes,
    doughnuts, bran cereals, popcorn.

Serve if desired:

- **Fats.** Butter or margarine, cream, cream sauce, salad oil,
crisp bacon, mayonnaise and salad dressing.

    Avoid: bacon grease, ham grease, highly spiced French
    dressing, gravy.

- **Soups.** Cream and vegetable soups made from foods that
are allowed. Strained cream soups may be made from most
vegetables that are not allowed.

    Avoid: commercially canned and frozen soups made from
    foods that are not allowed. Soups made with dried beans
    and peas, meat or chicken broth.

- **Sweets.** Moderate amounts of sugar, honey, jelly, seedless
jam, molasses, nuts, or fruits.

- **Desserts.** Plain desserts, such as custards, puddings, ice cream, sherbet, gelatin with allowed fruits, junket; angel food, sponge, and plain butter cake with simple frostings; plain cookies.

  Avoid: rich desserts, such as pies, rich cakes, cobblers, and other pastries; all other desserts containing nuts, coconut, and raisins.

- **Beverages.** Coffee, tea, or coffee substitutes.

  Avoid: alcohol, carbonated beverages.

- **Flavorings.** Allspice, chocolate, cinnamon, lemon juice, mace, paprika, salt, thyme, vinegar.

  Avoid: barbecue sauce, black pepper, chili pepper, chili sauce, cloves, horseradish, ketchup, mustard, nutmeg, nuts, olives, pickles, steak sauces.

FURTHER INSTRUCTIONS:

- It is very important to eat often, slowly, in a relaxed manner, and on schedule.
- Foods that cause your stomach to produce excess acid must be omitted or limited. These include alcohol, most spices, carbonated beverages, tea, coffee, and meat extracts, as well as tobacco.

Low-Sodium Diet

Be temperate with sodium intake at all times. Sodium is found not only in salt but also in baking soda, baking powder, many prepared foods, and commercial antacids that list sodium on the label. Please learn to read labels.

If you follow a low-sodium diet, prepare and serve all foods without salt, baking soda, or regular baking powder. Use salt-free butter or salt-free margarine. Limit your intake of bread (which contains salt and baking soda) to two slices a day. The only commercial canned vegetables or vegetable juices allowed are the low-sodium dietetic type.

Do not use laxatives or other medicines unless approved by your doctor (many laxatives are high in sodium). Use a salt substitute only if approved by your doctor.

Your diet should continue to be high in protein. Include each day one quart of milk, one egg, and one-half pound of lean meat or an alternative.

Serve every day:

- **Milk.** One quart milk, skim milk, or homemade buttermilk. One-half pint of milk contains 120 milligrams of sodium.

  Do not serve: more than the allowed amount of milk, commercial buttermilk, commercial chocolate milk, malted milk; "Dutch process" cocoa; instant cocoa mixes.

- **Eggs.** One only (includes eggs used in cooking). One egg contains 70 milligrams of sodium.

- **Meat or alternative.** Two large servings weighing four ounces each after being cooked (or each serving ½ by 3 by 4 inches). Four ounces of cooked meat, fish or poultry contain about 100 milligrams of sodium. Fresh, frozen, or canned low-sodium dietetic beef, chicken, duck, lamb, pork, quail, rabbit, tongue (fresh, cooked without salt), turkey, veal, liver (beef, calf, chicken, pork, with beef or calf liver allowed not more than once in two weeks). Fresh or canned low-sodium dietetic fish, except shellfish. Low-sodium dietetic ham, bacon, peanut butter. Unsalted cottage cheese. Dried beans or peas. Lemon juice, herbs, and spices may be used as seasonings. Meat or fish may be cooked with unsalted tomato juice, garlic, onion, or green pepper.

  Do not serve: brains; kidneys; canned, salted, or smoked meat, bacon, cold cuts, chipped or corned beef, frankfurters, ham, kosher meats, salt pork, sausage, smoked tongue, etc.; fresh fish fillets (sodium is used in processing them); shellfish such as crab, lobster, oysters, shrimp, etc.; cheeses except unsalted cottage cheese; salted peanut butter; meat extracts; bouillon.

- **Potato or alternative.** One serving or more. White or sweet potato; corn, dried beans or peas; macaroni, noodles, rice or spaghetti (all prepared without salt).

  Do not serve: potato chips, instant potatoes, potatoes fried in salty medium such as bacon fat. Sodium hydroxide is sometimes used in making hominy and grits.

- **Vegetables.** Two servings or more. Fresh, frozen or unsalted canned. One-quarter teaspoon of sugar added during the cooking period helps bring out the natural flavor of the vegetables. Also, adding one-quarter teaspoon herbs to three cups cooked vegetables improves flavor, as do lemon juice and vinegar. A good low-sodium mayonnaise or oil-and-vinegar dressing can be made by omitting salt from a standard recipe and substituting any of the spices or herbs allowed (see pages 82–83).

  Do not serve: regular canned vegetables and vegetable juices or the following vegetables in any form—artichokes, beet greens, beets, carrots, celery, kale, mustard or dandelion greens, sauerkraut, spinach, Swiss chard, white turnips, commercially frozen peas, corn or lima beans (sodium is used in processing them).

- **Fruits.** Two servings or more, of which one is an orange, half a grapefruit, the juice from either of these, or salt-free tomato or tomato juice. Use fresh, frozen, canned or dried fruit.

  Do not serve: crystallized or glazed fruit, maraschino cherries, dried or frozen fruits to which salt or other sodium compounds have been added (read labels).

- **Bread and cereal.** Only two servings of regular bread each day. The following may be eaten as desired: yeast breads and rolls made without salt; cooked unsalted cereals, such as instant and regular cream of wheat or rice, grits, oatmeal, puffed wheat, puffed rice, shredded wheat, homemade unsalted muffins, unsalted matzos.

Do not serve: canned biscuits, cornmeal, muffins, pancakes, or cakes made with mixes; products made with self-rising flour; quick cream of wheat or other quick-cooking cereals containing a sodium compound (read the label); graham crackers or any other crackers except low-sodium dietetic; pretzels.

Serve if desired:

- Unsalted butter or unsalted margarine.
- Soups made with allowed foods or unsalted canned soups.

Lack of salt doesn't make for a dull meal. The trick is to use the many flavorings and seasonings that help hide the lack of salt. Here are some tips on how to spice up your meals on a low-sodium diet.

FOR MEAT, POULTRY, FISH, GAME, EGGS

beef: allspice, bay leaf, dry mustard, lemon juice, nutmeg, onion, pepper, sage, tomato

pork: apples, applesauce, lemon juice, onion, parsley, pepper, pineapple, sage, thyme

fish: bay leaf, curry, dry mustard, ginger, lemon juice, onion, pepper, tomato

chicken and turkey: bay leaf, cranberry sauce, curry, ginger, lemon juice, onion, parsley, pepper, pineapple, sage, thyme

game: apples, lemon juice, onion, oranges, pepper, sage

eggs: dry mustard, jelly, onion, parsley, pepper, tomato

FOR VEGETABLES

asparagus: lemon juice

cabbage: dill seed, dry mustard, lemon juice, sugar

carrots: lemon juice, mint, nutmeg, parsley, sugar

corn: pimento, sugar, tomato

green beans: dill seed, lemon juice, onion, nutmeg, pepper sauce, sage, sugar

greens: pepper sauce
peas: lemon juice, mint, onion, parsley, pimento, sugar
potatoes: mace, nutmeg, onion, parsley, pimento
squash: ginger, mace, onion, sugar
tomatoes: bay leaf, celery, dill, onion, sage, sugar

OTHER SUGGESTIONS

Salt substitutes: Check with your doctor before using a salt substitute.

Lemon juice: Sprinkle lemon juice on meats, fish, salads and vegetables. You'll be pleasantly surprised at how much better they taste.

Meats: Barbecue meats are especially good when you leave out the salt. You can make your own barbecue sauce using any of these items: dry mustard, fat from fresh pork or unsalted butter, lemon juice, onion, pepper, salad oil, tomatoes (fresh or unsalted canned).

Bread: If you are allowed three slices of regular bread each day, you may want to mix one slice with your egg. The salt in the bread helps flavor the egg. French toast is a good way to combine bread and egg. You can mix your bread with vegetables, as in breaded tomatoes, or make into bread crumbs and sprinkle on top of a vegetable.

Things That Go Bump in the Night

Baby's Kicking

Morally, philosophically, and actually a baby is a living organism from the moment of conception. Shortly after a fertilized egg embeds in the womb, it begins to organize into recognizable structures, and once it is an established fetus, movements begin in the form of slight muscular contractions. This occurs sometime in the second month of pregnancy. Such movements soon begin to be more active and more powerful. However, the baby is so well cushioned in your uterus, is so completely surrounded by fluid, and is so small that it is usually not until sometime toward the end of the fourth month that movements are first felt. There is a great deal of variation in this time, and you should not be upset if movements are felt earlier or later. In many cases, movements are felt only slightly during the whole pregnancy and yet a perfectly normal child is delivered. Some babies are very active and some are not. But the degree of regular movement has only partial bearing on the actual health of the child.

Sometimes during normal pregnancy, movements *seem* to cease for days on end, and this may be a considerable source of anxiety. Actually, close observation will show movement to be present. The reasons for the cessation of awareness of them are unknown, but in almost all instances customary movements begin again spontaneously after a variable lapse, and the pregnancy goes on. You should, however, reassure yourself by going to the doctor's office and having a listen.

At times you may notice a rhythmic tapping inside your abdomen. This sort of movement is caused, we think, by contractions of the fetal diaphragm as it makes preliminary slight breathing efforts, similar to what happens when we hiccup.

Fetal movements are at first very faint and can best be described as a fluttering or shimmering sensation in the lower abdomen. Many times what are actually fetal movements are thought by the mother to be gas bubbles. After you have once experienced fetal movements, it is easier to recognize them again. Usually, then, you are able to feel your baby moving earlier in your second pregnancy than in your first.

Your baby may seem to be everywhere at one time, kicking your ribs and bladder simultaneously. How come? Well, your child is weightless inside you, like an astronaut in space or as you would be in saltwater. A baby can extend all four extremities and its head at the same time—and often does.

Many mothers ask, "Why is it that babies seem to become more active at night?" They pound on your bladder, put a foot into your ribs, hit your husband, and so forth. Well, baby does have regular sleep and wake periods and is often more active in the evening hours. As a matter of fact, some obstetricians are now asking mothers in certain high risk pregnancies to self-monitor their baby's movements during these active periods and to keep records of the activity rate. Under these circumstances movements should be noted and charted carefully, and any reduction in activity needs to be reported instantly. This information is undoubtedly of real value in assessing fetal well-being in certain at-risk situations.

Finally, fetal movements usually diminish shortly after labor begins. If you notice this do not become alarmed, unless, of course, you are monitoring the activity rate for special reasons, as noted.

Sex

Sex remains the single greatest and most gratifying form of interpersonal communication ever developed. This situation is not likely to change. Pregnancy does nothing to diminish this fact, but it may alter some of the circumstances and some of the ground rules. Herewith, in a question-and-answer format, are replies to many of your sex-during-pregnancy queries.

Is sexual intercourse permitted during pregnancy?

Like breathing and eating, sleeping and awakening, sexual intercourse is not only permissible but desirable during normal pregnancy. The only times it should not be part of your pregnant life are when you don't want to; when certain conditions, which will be discussed, make it dangerous; and finally, when it is no longer mutually rewarding. Being philosophical for the moment, I hope your married sexual goal has always been based on the giving of love to one another rather than receiving it, upon respecting one another's sexual wishes and upon making love rather than having sex. Also, hopefully, you have been able to explore each other's sexual anatomy and, through experimentation and mutual giving, you have learned that the more you practice, the better music you make. It is very important during the course of pregnancy, with all its emotional and physical changes, that these sexual aims be continued, further explored and mutually respected. It is a time for your husband to be considerate of the emotional and physical changes going on in your body. It's equally important for you to respect his continued desires and his need for you.

How long is sexual intercourse permissible?

Actually, you are asking how long is vaginal penetration permissible. Most frequently, vaginal penetration is the culmination of the sexual act or it plays a major role in most normal sexual encounters. Vaginal penetration may occur as long as it is mutually desirable and not painful and as long as it is not restricted specifically by your physician. Don't call *checkmate* because of the calendar or clock.

When is intercourse medically not permissible?

Generally, sexual intercourse (vaginal penetration) is restricted when vaginal bleeding is occurring at any stage of pregnancy for whatever reason, when there is severe vaginal infection that produces significant pain, when there is a history of incompetent cervical closure (see p. 225), when the membranes have ruptured, or when you are in labor.

What things may happen to make sex unenjoyable to me?

Local infections in the vagina; congestion of the vagina and pelvis, particularly late in pregnancy, especially if baby's head or presenting part is deep in your pelvis. At such times, other forms of mutual gratification can be explored.

After I have a climax, I notice menstrual-type cramping

that may last for an hour or so. Why does this happen? Is it dangerous?

When you have a sexual climax, the pituitary gland releases a hormone substance that makes your uterus contract. This is the source of your cramping in almost all instances and is of no danger to you.

Will such cramps start labor?

Almost never. If they did, most of us would not be here!

What position is the best for having sexual intercourse while I am pregnant?

As in riding a camel, there is no best position. There are only comfortable and mutually rewarding and satisfying positions. In early pregnancy there is very little change in your personal sexual habits. As the baby begins to occupy more of your abdomen, you will certainly want to experiment with positions that produce less abdominal pressure. Although such pressure is not necessarily harmful, it is neither rewarding nor pleasant. Other positions to be explored include sitting on top of your husband or having him penetrate you from behind. Do what comes comfortably. But do something.

Do any special preparations have to be made before having sex during pregnancy?

Sex is usually not prepared for very far in advance, which may be why you have to read this book now. Anyway, spontaneous lovemaking is generally more desirable. However, local vaginal hygiene with soap and water, if you wish, or douching with water or vinegar and water helps reduce the heavier secretions of pregnancy. Be sure to follow douching instructions mentioned in the discussion of hygiene on pages 49–50. Powders and perfumes on the vulva are fine, but aerosol sprays are not. A simple water-soluble lubricant, such as K-Y jelly, may be used if lubrication is desired, so long as it is not irritating to either of you. Incidentally, your husband's personal hygiene is important, since most vaginal infections during pregnancy are transmitted from your partner's fingers, penis, or mouth. Last but not least, in your sexual preparations, take the phone off the hook, lock the door and put K-Y jelly on the outside handle, hide the car, sedate the kids, and turn off the TV.

If vaginal penetration is uncomfortable because of pressure or irritation, are there alternatives we may use?

The most frequent alternatives are oral and anal intercourse or mutual masturbation. Again, if oral-genital relationships are desirable, personal hygiene is of vast importance. The instructions given on pages 47–50 should be followed closely. Insofar as anal intercourse is concerned, if vaginal penetration is uncomfortable at this stage, it is more than likely that anal penetration will be even more so. Also, anal penetration followed by vaginal penetration is out during pregnancy, as the risk of subsequent vaginal infection is too great. Late in pregnancy, mutual masturbation may be the only alternative. One more thing: Blowing into the vagina, a not uncommon sexual practice, is far too dangerous at this time.

I have a constant discharge from my breasts during pregnancy, which you have called colostrum, and this increases during sexual activity when my husband fondles and suckles my breasts. Is this harmful?

No, but the secretions may be bitter and he may wish to change this form of breast stimulation. He cannot hurt your nipples unless he bites them or has an oral infection.

When we have sexual intercourse, can we harm the baby?

Only in the conditions that are specified as we progress through this book.

Will sex make the water break?

In a normal pregnancy, no.

Will my climax change during pregnancy?

Your sexual drives are highly involved in your emotional life and are subject to vast changes under the psychological stress as well as the hormonal changes of pregnancy. Therefore, you may have a more deep and recurrent climax or you may have a less sustained climax. In the event that serious orgasmic failure occurs during pregnancy and continues afterward, it is important to seek counseling.

Will my husband's desires change?

They may. He, too, has emotional changes related to the pregnancy, which may be both good and bad. For instance, he may wish to overprotect you; he may fear the pregnancy; he may not want the changes that the baby produces in your body and in your daily and sexual life-style. There may be a thousand other subconscious reasons that interfere with his normal sexual drives.

If my husband and I develop a significant sexual problem during pregnancy or afterward, how can we best cope with this problem?

A serious sexual problem is not likely to arise if you have communicated freely as a couple in the past and have had no hangups or communication problems during the pregnancy. However, should a sexual problem of significant magnitude occur while you are pregnant, there are resources available to help you cope. First, of course, discuss the difficulty with your partner. Should this avenue fail or not be open to you, you should next talk with your obstetrician. Only a few doctors are trained to manage these problems themselves and usually in a busy practice do not have time to explore them with you in sufficient depth. However, if yours is a patient-oriented doctor, trained in sexual counseling—and they are on the increase— you may be able to get sufficient help. Otherwise you should ask your doctor who might best counsel you further. There are many good sex therapists and clinical psychologists available in today's market. Your husband should accompany you, but even if he doesn't, you should visit such a counselor on your own.

Just out of curiosity, are persons who have had their sex changed by surgery able to reproduce?
No; they can breed plants and animals, but not each other.

Showing

Somewhere between the third and the fifth month, one of your prime assets temporarily disappears. Your wisp of a waist begins to expand rapidly, and the flatland below it now has a perceptible bulge. This anatomical phenomenon is known as showing. For numerous reasons, it occurs at different times in different women. The abdomen of a mother who has previously borne children stretches more readily, so that showing is more likely to occur early in her pregnancy. Also, basic anatomy makes a difference. For instance, those of you with long, deep abdomens may hardly show at all during pregnancy. The size of the uterus is another controlling factor. This, in turn, depends upon the baby's weight, the number of babies present, and the amount of surrounding amniotic fluid.

All these factors plus a few others contribute to determining when you lose the battle of the bulge. And whenever this might be, it has no bearing on whether your pregnancy is normal. All it determines is when you have to get out of slacks and into sacks!

A Simple Matter of Elimination

Constipation

We spend the early years of our children's lives training them to hold on to things till we can get them on the potty. They spend the rest of their years trying to get on the potty when it is convenient rather than when the urge comes. The result of this constant colonic conflict is constipation and the consequent sale of millions of dollars' worth of laxatives, enemas, and hemorrhoid preparations.

Constipation, a prevalent problem in our society, is even more common during pregnancy. Functional changes in the intestines as well as pressure on the lower bowel and rectum invite constipation, and even worse, the tendency toward constipation combined with rectal pressure predisposes to the formation of hemorrhoids and may produce rectal burning, itching, and pain as well as bleeding. Constipation should be avoided by:

- immediate response to the desire to have a bowel movement
- eating fruits, raw or cooked, that have a laxative effect
- eating roughage—leafy vegetables and prepared cereals, particularly bran
- drinking plenty of fluids

The presence of regular, soft bowel movements helps greatly in the prevention of hemorrhoids. It is important to avoid straining after the initial bowel evacuation even if you feel there is still material to be passed. This feeling of fullness may well be due to engorgement of the rectal veins, and straining only serves to engorge them further, bringing them to the outside and producing clinical hemorrhoids. The treatment of hemorrhoids, when they do occur, should be individualized, and you should call your doctor for proper care.

Mild laxatives may be used during pregnancy; milk of magnesia is probably the mildest and the safest. Before submitting yourself to this, however, you might try using prepared bulk agents such as Metamucil. In a harmless, nonirritating way these often give your bowel movement the bulk needed to avoid constipation. More drastic medications must be ordered by your doctor. Further, it is safe to take an enema during pregnancy; indeed, it is safer than some laxatives. Disposable enema packages can be purchased at your drugstore.

Incidentally, the iron in your prenatal vitamin-mineral supplement may produce a black bowel movement that is constipating. You may have to get your iron some other way. Ask your doctor. More rarely, iron may give you diarrhea, and iron will have to be given in some other form.

Habits

Good habits are proper eating and sleeping, exercise, scrupulous personal hygiene, responsible living, speaking the truth, and so on. Bad habits are what we are saddled with and sometimes constitute our way of life. We are all creatures of habit, and generally your habits are well formed by the time you conceive. Some affect pregnancy and some don't.

Tobacco

There are two legal social poisons: tobacco and alcohol. Cigarette smoking is a very nasty, expensive, dangerously filthy habit, as anyone who doesn't smoke will be glad to tell you. It has now been proved beyond a reasonable doubt that smoking during pregnancy is hazardous to the well-being of the fetus and to the health of a newborn baby and its future development, as well as being hazardous to the mother herself. For women who do smoke—and this constitutes 33 percent of women of childbearing age—pregnancy can be double trouble. While it is one of the most important times to stop smoking, it is also one of the most difficult times to do so. A pregnant woman who smokes twenty cigarettes per day inhales tobacco smoke, with its one thousand diverse and poisonous chemicals, 11,000 times during an average pregnancy, and she may spend 10 percent of her waking day smoking.

What are the fetal effects of this immense problem?

- Impaired fetal growth and development. It has been shown clearly and beyond doubt that infants of pregnant mothers who smoke are born smaller, with significantly lower IQ scores, increased occurrences of reading disorders and evidence of the minimal brain dysfunction syndrome. These observations suggest that the fetal central nervous system is impaired as a result of maternal smoking.

- Increased risk of spontaneous abortion and intrauterine fetal death and even SIDS (sudden infant death syndrome) related directly to the level of maternal smoking activity. For instance, the incidence of fetal loss in women who smoke more than one pack per day is 35 percent greater than that for women who smoke less than that amount.

- Adverse maternal effect. There is an increased incidence of serious and potentially lethal complications in the expectant mother who smokes. Premature separation of the placenta occurs significantly more frequently in smokers than in nonsmokers, and the rate of occurrence increases significantly as the rate of smoking increases. Abnormal location of the placenta is greater in women who smoke. These facts, of course, are in addition to the long-term effects of smoking on the pregnant mother's health. These include chronic bronchitis, emphysema and lung cancer, cardiovascular disease, atherosclerosis, increased risk of bladder cancer, and, finally, peptic ulcer disease. The mortality rate in these women is 30–80 percent greater than in matched nonsmokers. It is unfortunate that at this time cigarette and tobacco advertising is being more and more directed to young women, and their share of the cigarette market is increasingly significant. This advertising trend began about twenty years ago, and the mortal harvest is now coming in. In several of our states and in all of Canada, cancer of the lungs now kills more women than cancer of the breast.

It is important, then, that you attempt to eliminate or reduce smoking during your pregnancy. There are clinics in almost any community, many of them free, that will work to assist you in this vastly important program. The new nicotine gums, incidentally, still put nicotine into your circulation and into your unborn child's circulation.

If you wish any proof of what effect your smoking is having upon you and your baby, your doctor can very easily draw a carbon monoxide level from your blood. Remember that the level in your unborn child is greater than that which you exhibit. And finally, remember that while you're nursing, sidestream smoking from your exhaled breath begins your baby's poisoning, too.

If you share a room in the hospital with a nonsmoker or a light smoker, it is not good manners nor is it fair for you or your guests to fill the room with smoke during visiting hours or at any other time. More and more hospitals are banning cigarette smoking altogether, by patients, doctors, visitors, personnel—everyone. This kind of ban is likely to become more widespread in coming years.

Alcohol

Although many expectant mothers who are accustomed to drinking alcohol may wish to continue doing so during pregnancy, they often lose their taste for it in the earlier months and lose their tolerance for it in the later months. More important, as we shall now see, alcohol has profound effects upon pregnancy. Whether or not your taste for alcohol continues unchanged during pregnancy, you must alert yourself to the facts demonstrated in the vast accumulation of literature showing the harmful effects that alcohol can have upon fetal development. Indeed, fetal alcohol syndrome is a clearly defined entity, and babies born out of this environment typically have a flat midface, a short upturned nose, a low nasal bridge, and smaller than average eyes. Worse still, many major abnormalities combine with this typical facial appearance. These include growth retardation both in the uterus and out, microcephaly (small head), delayed learning abilities, and disturbed motor function.

Of equal significance are the obstetrical problems that alcohol ingestion provokes. Thus, abortion and intrauterine fetal death are common. Infants of alcoholic mothers may be born suffering from acute alcohol withdrawal symptoms severe enough to be life threatening.

Although the case against modest alcohol consumption during pregnancy *may* be slightly overstated, it certainly should be respected, and no more than one ounce of hard liquor, four ounces of wine or one can of beer should be consumed in any one pregnant day.

The chronic alcoholic presents a disastrous picture during pregnancy. According to a recent study, she has a 45- to 50-percent chance of producing a severely malformed infant. Because of this risk of congenital malformation and all the other associated dangers, a chronic alcoholic should avoid pregnancy; if it takes place, therapeutic abortion should be seriously considered. In many practicing obstetricians' opinion, this sad disease is, in fact, a good, sufficient, and compelling reason for an abortion procedure.

Heavy and Hard Stuff

There is significant evidence now that marijuana, LSD, cocaine, and most of the other powerful stimulants and drugs that are illegal to possess and use have very significant and damaging fetal effects. Mind-expanding drugs such as LSD are not only dangerous for the user but have been shown to produce profound destructive fetal effects. Heroin addicts deliver addicted babies who die after delivery from withdrawal symptoms if the symptoms go unrecognized. Over half such babies are premature. A recent legal decision found an addict mother guilty of child neglect after her baby was born addicted. Methadone-treated mothers usually have normal-size babies, but it is much more difficult to withdraw these babies than those who are addicted to heroin. Many fail to make it. Marijuana, it is now established, is more potent as a fetal damager than tobacco.

The poisons in the preceding paragraphs, whether acceptable or unacceptable socially, are not to be recommended during pregnancy or at any other time, though some of them apparently must be tolerated. If you wish to expand your mind, *thinking* is a simple, inexpensive, rewarding, and successful way to do so.

Sleeping

Sleeping is not a habit but a physiological need around which we form many habits. Eight hours is the prescribed average amount of sleep during a twenty-four-hour period. But there is a tremendous variation in personal needs. In the early months of pregnancy, more sleep is required and an afternoon nap is very beneficial. If you cannot manage a nap, retire early enough in the evening to get the rest you need.

Your sleep will be interrupted in the last months by a number of little things. First of all, the creature inside you seems to make all major adjustments at night. Second, everything aches in every part of your body, and cramps tantalize your legs as dawn approaches. Finally, your bladder capacity is about the same as that of the fuel tank of a toy truck.

Sometimes, in fact oftentimes, you may have a real problem just getting to sleep, let alone staying there. Again, sad to relate, there isn't even a mild sedative, used however infrequently, that is cleared for use in pregnancy. Quite likely some agents that are helpful in sleepless situations, when taken correctly, are going to be proved harmless to expectant mothers and completely formed babies. Yet in our adversary society no one will absolutely clear them. These drugs being therefore suspect, few physicians are likely to risk prescribing them. So you are a prisoner of insomnia and can only dream of sleep—if you ever get to dream!

Fascinating Facts

▷ Consider this dietary advice, which was given to pregnant women about a hundred years ago.

Eat only twice daily. . . . Excessive indulgence in food has hurried more people to the grave than war, famine, pestilence, and alcohol combined . . . its ravages are ceaseless; from year to year it pursues its work of destruction without pause for interruption. . . . It wastes not only cities and provinces but rioting throughout the whole broad world, it spreads disease and death amongst all classes, ages, sexes, and conditions—maidens and matrons—infants and children—the feeble and robust—all are swept indiscriminately into the grave by this fell destroyer. [Wilhelmine D. Schott, *Health Hints to Women* (New York: Charles P. Somerby, 1883.)]

▷ An improper diet is actually *more* dangerous to your baby than are moderate smoking and drinking! But all of them are harmful.

DIARY

My Third Month

Problems ————————————————————

Medications ————————————————————

————————————————————

————————————————————

Travel ————————————————————

————————————————————

————————————————————

Diet problems ————————————————————

————————————————————

————————————————————

Baby moved? When? ————————————————————

What's going on in the world? ————————————————————

————————————————————

————————————————————

————————————————————

What's going on in my life? ————————————————————

————————————————————

————————————————————

————————————————————

My thoughts and feelings ————————————————————

————————————————————

————————————————————

————————————————————

Doctor's appointment ————————————————————

Questions To Ask

_____

_____

_____

_____

_____

_____

_____

_____

_____

_____

_____

_____

_____

_____

_____

_____

_____

_____

_____

_____

_____

_____

_____

_____

_____

CHAPTER FOUR

MY FOURTH
LUNAR MONTH

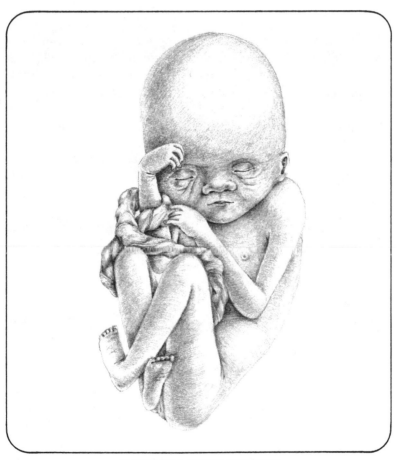

FOURTH LUNAR MONTH

The fourth lunar month is a rather quiet time in your pregnancy. You've learned to swim, as it were, but haven't hit the deep water yet, and so it will give us a chance to discuss certain complications along the way. Though some of these problems are not too pleasant, it is your need to know and my obligation to tell you about them. But first let's see just where you are.

Your uterus has now risen into the abdomen, and you can probably begin to feel it protruding gently just above the pubic bone at the bottom of your tummy. Your baby weighs only three ounces (85 grams), is sixteen centimeters (6½ inches) long, and moving very actively. You have already had to adjust your clothing, and you will probably have to adjust your automobile seatbelt and seat. Although completely formed, your baby is still susceptible to damage or injury from a large number of substances and activities, all of which are being dealt with as we go along. You may wonder how, with so many possible means of being damaged, any child could arrive on earth in good health and completely developed. I tend to agree with you. But nature, with its marvelous ability to overprotect, scan, and adapt, guards your baby much better than you would ever imagine. Even so, remember our original premise: Nature, if left alone, is relentless in its performance and so doesn't always do what *we* consider best.

Vaginal Infections

Another question-and-answer session.

Vaginal Discharge and Vaginitis

I have a heavy vaginal discharge now that I am pregnant. Is this common, and what can be done for it?
Since there is a great deal of congestion in the pelvis and all the surrounding tissues, it is very, very common for you to have an increase in vaginal secretions during pregnancy. However, such discharge should not be irritating or produce any itching, redness, or swelling. Neither should it produce discomfort during intercourse. If any of these occur, a vaginal infection is probably present.

The normal vaginal secretion may be malodorous or unpleasant to you because it contains lactic acid, which is always present in the vagina to some degree. Lactic acid is made from sugar found in the cells that line the vagina, reacting with certain bacteria normally present in this area.

To reduce these normal secretions, you may douche, as previously mentioned, with gravity-flow equipment. You should not douche with syringe bulb devices while you are pregnant since you may inadvertently introduce the syringe into the cervix, which can produce disastrous results. You may use clear water as your douching liquid or a standard vinegar and water combination. Do not use medicated douches without specific instructions.

How far into pregnancy may I douche?
You may douche until it is no longer comfortable to insert the douche nozzle into the vagina or unless bleeding is present or follows douching. Your doctor may not want you to douche at all. Ask.

What about the use of sprays and deodorants during pregnancy in order to control vaginal odors?

Douching, soap and water, and body powder are the best deodorants. Sprays are for setting hair, killing insects, waxing cars, and polluting the atmosphere.

With such a heavy vaginal discharge, how can I tell if I have an infection?

If you develop a vaginal infection, there are certain unmistakable changes. First, the amount of discharge will likely increase. Second, it will probably change in character to either frothy yellowish or thick and white. Third, your vagina, its entrance, and the surrounding areas will become irritated, red, swollen, and itching, and sex will be as comfortable as lying on a bed of coals.

What are the most common vaginal infections that occur during pregnancy?

In order of frequency: yeast (monilia, fungus, candida), trichomonas, and bacterial (including gonorrhea).

Yeast Infections

Why are yeast infections the most common?

Changes in the moisture and acidity of the vagina and the presence of free urine sugar, plus the prevalence of yeast organisms in our environment all contribute to make this the most common vaginal infection during pregnancy.

What is a yeast infection?

A yeast infection is one caused by a parasitic fungus that lives mainly on human tissue. It is called *Candida albicans* and is found in the vagina but occurs on other parts of the body and can be carried by men in various parts of their body.

104

Is it a venereal disease?

No. It can be contracted from tubs, toilet seats, clothing, and a variety of other sources.

How are yeast infections treated?

It is hard to completely eradicate yeast infections during pregnancy. Control may be obtained, however, by the use of vaginal suppositories and creams specifically designed to destroy *Candida albicans* growth. Suppositories come with an inserter, but it would be better to insert such medication with your fingers and wash carefully afterward. Creams must be inserted with an applicator. You probably should use the suppositories or creams for at least a week, even if your symptoms have disappeared. The only symptom that does not disappear is the discharge, since the medications have to run back out. However, the irritation, redness, and swelling should melt away. You may very well become reinfected during pregnancy, so keep extra medication on hand.

What can I do to prevent or control recurrence?

Avoid the common sources of infection. Take showers instead of tub baths and wash your bottom very thoroughly with soap and water. If, however, you prefer taking tub baths, rinse the tub well with chlorine bleach and water before you get in and after you get out. Put toilet paper around any toilet seat you sit on, wear cotton panties and boil them before wearing them again or get the new self-adhesive minipads that are available commercially. Avoid pantyhose, even those with a cotton crotch. Boiled pantyhose end up cobwebs! If infections flare up after intercourse, be sure your husband does not have a yeast infection. He may carry yeast under the glands of his foreskin if he is not circumcised, in his groin if he has "jockey itch," on his fingers or his feet. Have him clean up before sex. Wearing a condom may be helpful. All these things help prevent recurrence, but the complete eradication of yeast infections will often not be possible until after your pregnancy is over.

Can yeast infections affect my baby?

Yes. If you have an active yeast infection when you deliver, your baby may get a yeast infection in its mouth called thrush. This is not dangerous and can be simply treated by your pediatrician.

Trichomonas

What are the symptoms of a trichomonas infection?

Usually they are about the same as for a yeast infection, except that the discharge is more likely to be a thin, yellowish, frothy discharge with a great deal of irritation and itching. It is less common during pregnancy.

Can it be treated during pregnancy?

Yes, though the most satisfactory treatment for trichomonas infections, an oral tablet taken by both husband and wife, has not been proved safe for use during pregnancy. However, there are suppositories that can control the infection throughout the pregnancy, and if reinfection occurs after delivery, the oral method of treatment may be used.

How can I control this infection?

By using the same restrictive techniques that were described for yeast infections.

Is there any danger to the baby from trichomonas infections?

No.

Where do trichomonas organisms live?

In the vagina, the surrounding tissues, the rectum, and the male prostate gland.

Is trichomonas a venereal disease?

Not necessarily. Trichomonas organisms live on toilet seats, in tubs, and on douching equipment for some period of time and can occasionally be transmitted by contact with them.

Bacterial

Are bacterial infections common during pregnancy?

Generally they are not. The most common one is *Gardnerella vaginalis*, which is not dangerous but is difficult to treat while you are pregnant. The most dangerous bacterial infection in pregnancy is gonorrhea.

How common is gonorrhea during pregnancy?

There are no reliable statistics at present related to the frequency of gonorrhea during pregnancy, but it is increasing rapidly because of our changing social customs and the marked increase in freedom of both sexual and social intercourse.

What symptoms does gonorrhea produce?

Sometimes very few, if any. There generally is a yellowish discharge and occasionally some irritation.

How can it be diagnosed?

By a high index of suspicion by your physician, and by culture taken from either the cervix, the urethra, the rectum, or all three.

What is the treatment?

The best treatment during pregnancy is a combination of penicillin and certain other drugs designed to destroy the bacteria.

Is there any danger to the baby if I have gonorrhea?

Only at the time of delivery. Your baby may develop a form of gonorrhea in its eyes which can produce blindness. This is largely preventable, however, with observation and care by your doctor.

Is there any danger to other children in my household, particularly female children, of picking up any of these

infections that you have described?

There is a very slight risk. If, however, you have mature daughters, they may pick up yeast or trichomonas from your toilet or bathtub. They will then have to undergo the same treatment you did.

Herpes

Are there any other vaginal infections that may occur in pregnancy?

There are others of importance, but only two of them need to be mentioned now. One is herpes virus II, related to the virus that causes cold sores about the mouth (herpes I). Genital herpes virus is sexually transmitted and is characterized by very painful small, shallow ulcers at the entrance of the vagina.

Can these be treated?

There are certain local medications that can be helpful in treatment, but virus diseases are hard to treat anywhere in the body and, in general, immunization is required for prevention. Unfortunately, there is not as yet a vaccine for herpes virus.

Can herpes virus damage my baby?

Very definitely. If you have such an infection at delivery, it can be transmitted to your child. It would be wise to be delivered by cesarean section. Your doctor will know this.

This is frightening. Is the disease common?

Until recently it has been rare, but, again, because of present sexual freedoms, it is increasing in frequency. Be sure to report to your doctor if you have painful ulcers in or around your vaginal entrance.

T. mycoplasmosis

You said that there were two vaginal infections of importance.

Yes, the other one is an unusual bacteria called *T. mycoplasmosis.* It is very difficult to culture and identify this bacteria, even in the best bacteriology laboratories.

What are its symptoms?

Just about none. You may have a slight vaginal discharge or some irritation at the neck of the bladder (the urethra), but you may have no symptoms at all.

What are its dangers to my pregnancy?

There are two, maybe more. First, *T. mycoplasmosis* is found very frequently in the genitals of sterile couples and it is believed to be a significant factor in causing infertility. Second, it is apparently a cause of early spontaneous abortion.

Will it cause anything else?

Not that we know of at this time.

How can it be discovered?

By a high index of suspicion on the part of your physician, particularly when he is studying infertility or repeated spontaneous abortions; by cultures that are very difficult to obtain and read; and, more easily, by certain blood tests.

Can *T. mycoplasmosis* be treated?

It responds to certain antibiotics, and the results of treatment can be checked by a drop in your blood sensitivity level.

Before leaving this section, I must say that there are other viral and bacterial infections in the vagina and cervix that can affect conception and pregnancy. You will probably be reading about cytomegalovirus (in fact, see p. 115), chlamydia, hepatitis B group, and group B streptococcus. Even *P. pubis,* the common pubic crab, is making a comeback! Finally, another vulvovaginal infection that is on the comeback trail is the common venereal wart, condylomata accuminata. This is caused by a sexually transmitted papilloma virus. However, venereal warts are easily treated and offer no danger that we are aware of to your baby. They occur singly or in clusters, generally on the vulva, at the vaginal entrance, and around the rectum. They look like warts, may be pinpoint or gigantic in size, and often become infected and irritating. But your doctor knows how to treat them. Incidentally, condylomata are now further incriminated in certain premalignantlike changes in the cervix.

We are just beginning to accumulate data on other "new" vaginal infections. We are trying to learn to control them and to assure you and your baby a safer journey. But, as you can see, all these infections are sex related, and also, as you can see—and as the press reminds us—they are expanding, multiplying, and diversifying at a frightening rate. Alas, sexual freedom is a myth. Disregarding the social, moral, and reproductive problems it spawns, the disastrous epidemics that follow are propelling us toward sexual myopia.

The *Torch* Syndrome

The *Torch* Syndrome is an acronym for a group of infectious processes all known to be or highly suspected of being damaging to babies either in the uterus, at birth, or during their early life. Let's see what the word is built upon.

T—toxoplasmosis
O—others
    hepatitis B
    B streptococcus
    influenza, mumps and chicken pox (varicella)
    others as yet unknown
R—rubella (German measles)

C—cytomegalovirus
H—herpes virus II

Most of these infectious processes are mentioned elsewhere in this book; why, then, are they grouped together here?

- Infections in newborns associated with these agents are generally indistinguishable one from the other except by very special tests.
- Infection in newborns is often inapparent and late to appear, but it can cause long-term serious damage.
- Most important, infection in the mother is usually clinically inapparent or simply passed off as the flu or mono or "some virus."
- Treatment is difficult for most of these, but prevention and treatment are improving.
- Grouped together, they represent a significant problem that needs medical and social attention.
- While it has been estimated that these infections involve as many as 5 to 15 percent of all pregnancies, at most only 1 to 2 percent of the affected fetuses are structurally damaged as a result.

Infants who are afflicted by any one of the *Torch* infections may have a variety of abnormalities, depending upon when the infection strikes. If it occurs in early pregnancy, that is, the first trimester, the damage generally involves the heart, eyes, neurological system, or blood-forming system. Infections sustained later in the pregnancy generally produce more subtle problems, such as failure to thrive, low birth rate, perceptual handicaps, mental retardation, and certain other more rare conditions.

As noted, taken alone, these infections don't represent a big problem, but grouped together, they are considerably more compelling. Each will be covered here, but only briefly. For more detailed information consult your own doctor.

Toxoplasmosis

This organism is present in the droppings of cats that probably originally became diseased by eating infected rodents. Toxoplasmosis is also present in uncooked meat, particularly pork, although this is rare in the United States. And finally, of course, it is in human blood—the blood of those infected by cats or food. It is transmitted from these sources by a variety of mechanisms. Symptoms are just like those of flu or mononucleosis, but toxoplasmosis can cause abortions, stillbirths, prematurity, low birth rate for pregnancy duration, and infectious and developmental problems in later life. Drugs used to treat this disease have not generally been cleared by the Food and Drug Administration for use during pregnancy. However, a form of sulfa drug (sulfadiazine) is effective and can generally be used before the last two months of pregnancy. The best protection from toxoplasmosis is as follows:

- Avoid cats. If you own one, do not handle its litter box no matter whether it is an indoor or an outdoor cat. Don't even let the cat lick your face. Unless you love the cat more than your expected child, lend it to a friend.
- Cook meat thoroughly.
- This is probably redundant and ridiculous to suggest, but avoid a blood transfusion unless, of course, it is lifesaving.

Your obstetrician probably will test you for toxoplasmosis immunity when you first see him or her and again if you should develop a suspicious virallike infection. Although you cannot have medicine, your child can be treated successfully after birth if found to be infected. Remember, in order to infect a baby, all these *Torch* infections have to cross the placenta. They don't often make it across, so the baby is generally protected. It *must* be watched, though.

Hepatitis B

This virus can be transmitted in many ways, for example, by blood transfusion, needle puncture, tattooing, ear piercing, contamination in a hospital, contamination by human feces or blood, and even by sexual intercourse (through contact with contaminated saliva, semen, or feces). The later in pregnancy that hepatitis is acquired, the more likely is the child to acquire it and thus possibly become a carrier. Symptoms may be specific or they may be like any of the others in this *Torch* family. Passive immunization can be given, and fortunately a vaccine is available now to protect susceptible and exposed individuals.

Group B Beta Hemolytic Streptococcus

Little is yet known about the effects on the fetus of this sexually transmitted bacteria. The symptoms consist only of a vaginal infection. A baby would be infected at delivery, particularly in premature rupture of the membranes (see PROM, chapter 8). The treatment during pregnancy is local antibiotics. Systemic antibiotics may be used at term and in labor.

Influenza and Mumps

The evidence is unclear but growing that there appears to be a relationship between Asian influenza in particular and later severe blood disorders in a child exposed within the uterus. Vaccines for influenza and mumps are available. During pregnancy, avoid public exposure in epidemic areas.

Varicella (chickenpox)

This is perhaps the most infectious of all common virus diseases, with an attack rate of more than 90 percent of those who are exposed. Interestingly, this herpes virus is in the same family as

113

herpes virus II, which has been a front-page, highly distorted attention-getter in recent times. Chickenpox occurs in only 1 of 7,500 pregnancies, and the diagnosis is usually made by clinical signs on the skin. Although there is some very slight risk of the mother ending up with deadly varicella pneumonia, this is fortunately exceedingly rare. The fetal damage lies among those that are mentioned earlier along with scarring of the skin surfaces, small scars on extremities, and greatly increased susceptibility to future infections. There is no treatment for this viral infection.

Rubella (German measles)

Sadly, this disease could be wiped from the face of the earth, just as smallpox and polio are about to be. All that is needed is childhood vaccination of everyone—except the poor child who has already contracted it in the uterus of his unvaccinated, infected mother. He or she is born immune for life—and may well be deaf or worse for life. Here are a few simple facts:

- Do not ever get vaccinated against rubella during pregnancy.
- Rubella is most dangerous in early pregnancy as far as deformities are concerned. Thus, if the disease is contracted in the first three or four months, abortion, if morally acceptable, is the treatment of choice.
- Your children can be vaccinated while you are pregnant.
- There is no need to immunize a child who has contracted the disease in utero.
- If you have never been vaccinated or are not immune (your obstetrician can tell you), then get vaccinated before you leave the hospital after delivery. You will not infect your newborn, even if you breast-feed. And you are not likely to get pregnant for the next two months.
- Do not get pregnant sixty days subsequent to vaccination.
- We still don't know if revaccination is necessary.

- If you have neglected your children's vaccination program, make sure your daughters are tested and, if necessary, vaccinated at the time they go for their premarital blood test. This, incidentally, is already the law in at least one state.
- Report to your doctor if you have fever, runny eyes, sore throat, swollen glands, and a rash. It might be one of the other *Torch* disorders—by now I am sure you are so spooked you will report anything—but the other disorders are equally or more damaging.

Cytomegalovirus (CMV)

The CMV category includes a group of virus families that may cause a mild general illness in the host and, in women, may reside in the cervix for long periods of time. It may well be and probably is sexually transmitted. It is more common in lower socioeconomic groups. Unfortunately, not much is understood about this virus family or how to control it. An unborn child may acquire the virus at birth or across the placenta, which is worse. The affected infant has growth problems, hearing defects, and a lower IQ. There is no way of testing for this disease in any regular laboratory; neither can your doctor help you. Soon, thank goodness, there will be a routine test for newborns that will indicate the presence of CMV as well as many other *Torch* disorders.

The only treatment of CMV is highly experimental and cannot be used during pregnancy. Vaccines for CMV pose special dangers, necessitating prolonged study, but they may be available someday.

Herpes Virus II

This ever-increasing sexually transmitted virus was discussed earlier along with other vaginal infections. It rarely produces systemic symptoms, but the distribution and character of the shallow painful ulcers are almost enough to make a diagnosis from; a smear and culture of any open ulcer can be absolutely diagnostic. Only local treatment is used and it is of little help. A vaccine may be on the way. Your doctor may well decide to deliver you by cesarean section and will know what method to use.

Regarding these *Torch* diseases, remember, if you will, that they will yield to further study; some are already under control to some extent, as you have seen. Since your life during pregnancy and delivery is no longer in jeopardy, science is now concentrating on your baby's well-being. Great effort is being expended to bring these and other problems of childbearing and infancy to their knees. Let's not find any new ones!

The High-Risk Pregnancy

In the beginning of the book I said that never was there a better time to be pregnant and that pregnancy itself is not a disease. But in each succeeding chapter I open another can of worms and provide you with something else to worry about! I tell you, for instance, that the chance for a certain complication is 12 percent, and for the next one, 8 percent; for the next, 20 percent; and so on—when you add it all up for yourself, you find there is a 150 percent chance that something terrible is going to get you or your baby—or both of you—before it's all over! And so your worry gets greater and you wonder why I still expect you to come through smiling, smelling flowers all the way.

Well, you can do it. Ninety-nine percent of what goes on is good news. But no one would read it if I didn't report the bad news along with it!

All this serves as a bridgehead to introduce the subject of high-risk obstetrics—pregnancies that have a greater risk of adverse outcome for mother, child, or both. All obstetricians can and do manage these problems, but in many tertiary care centers (see Regionalized Care in the Glossary) they are dealt with by perinatologists—specialists in maternal-fetal medicine who concentrate their efforts on obstetrical risk situations (see p. 194).

Who actually is at risk? Well, very young and very old expectant mothers, diabetics, hypertensives, cardiacs, the obese, those with renal disease, and others. There are, of course, many categories of problems that constitute high risk, and indeed a normal pregnancy can suddenly become a high-risk one when, for instance, hypertension of pregnancy imposes itself (see chapter 6). Finally, there are areas of high-risk obstetrics that are almost experimental; that is, some of them have never really occurred before. An example of this would be pregnancy following coronary artery bypass surgery or following organ transplants or complicated by AIDS. And just such cases are beginning to appear. In subsequent chapters certain high-risk situations will be dealt with separately and in more detail. These include such areas as diabetics, hypertension of pregnancy, pregnancy in the elderly and very young and so on. It will be impossible, however, to detail the management of every one of these disorders that complicate pregnancy.

What we must know to deal with a difficulty is the effect of the disorder on pregnancy and the effect of pregnancy on the disorder. Armed with this information, doctors adapt the pregnancy management to the risk problem. The outcome is not always good. About the expectant mother, as you already know, we are pretty secure; the pregnancy itself, however, may be touch-and-go in many instances. Remember that most high risk pregnancies represent individuals who in the past could never conceive or carry a pregnancy.

Management

Each high-risk pregnancy, then, is managed individually. Those at high risk are seen by their doctors more frequently during pregnancy, and special tests and procedures are called into play at varying time intervals. Perhaps an example would make the idea of a management program a little more clear. Suppose, for instance, we are dealing with a pregnancy in which the expectant mother is hypertensive to a moderately severe degree. In the initial visit there is a complete evaluation of the mother's cardiovascular capacity, its functional reserve, and kidney reserve and function. Special dietary, weight, and exercise instructions are given, along with signs to be watched for that might indicate impending trouble. The pregnancy is followed very closely, and even if all is going well, beginning at around the twenty-eighth week, visits to the doctor would probably be scheduled for every two weeks or perhaps even every week. The doctor would be looking for evidence of increasing hypertension or for the addition of hypertension of pregnancy to the existing problem, for evidence of potential heart failure or kidney failure, and, finally but of equal importance, for evidence of fetal health and well-being. Doctors would be looking for evidence of intrauterine growth retardation or placental failure. The nonstress test and the stress test and ultrasound monitor, the biophysical profile—all will closely monitor the progress of the pregnancy (see Appendix). As full term approaches, evidence of fetal maturity will be sought as well as any further evidence of fetal distress. At the opportune time for both mother and child, delivery will be effected by the method calculated to cause the least trauma to both.

This is but one brief example of high-risk pregnancy management, and it is admittedly abbreviated and incomplete. However, it may serve to give you an idea of some of the problems involved in obstetrical risk management.

Usually following the delivery of a high-risk pregnancy and particularly if there has been fetal distress, the newborn is transferred to an intensive care nursery where pediatricians and neonatologists, in a relatively new branch of medicine, will watch over the child. Regardless, all our well-planned programs sometimes fail and we have a bad outcome. We are, however, gaining rapidly in preventing fetal loss and improving the quality of life for the little survivor. It is also true, no matter how far we advance, that there will always be new and distant barricades to attack and strike down. You, the undelivered, stand at the old barricade and may fear the crossing. We, for the most part, stand on the other side and have the confidence and the knowledge that we can get you through. That's our part of the covenant, and that's enough philosophy.

Medicines and Drugs

We have already talked in broad general terms in chapter 1 about the risks of medications and drugs during pregnancy. Total avoidance of drugs during pregnancy is a defensible but hardly a realistic position. Sometimes it is absolutely necessary to use some agent during pregnancy, but most times it is not. Remember these key points:

- About 90 percent of pregnant women take some medication other than their vitamins.
- Some 10 percent take ten to nineteen other drugs, and 6 percent actually take more than twenty. That's a fact!
- Forty percent of these medicines are taken in the first trimester.
- At the end of one year, 5 percent of all newborns have demonstrated developmental abnormalities that are probably drug related. This figure, however, includes the abuse of alcohol.
- Some medications are known to accumulate in the baby's circulation. Sometimes the accumulation is much in excess of that in the mothers.

The most dangerous agents ingested during pregnancy are called teratogens. Teratogens produce physical deformities in the fetus. Others, called clastogens, can in a toxic way damage the fetus without necessarily making visible or detectable structural alterations. Here is a list of *some* of the major identifiable medications and drugs, both prescription and over-the-counter, that have known destructive fetal effects.

Prescription Drugs

TERATOGENS

Thalidomide (a sedative, not available now in the U.S.)
Dilantin (a cerebral relaxant)
warfarin (an anticoagulant)
folic acid antagonist (generally present in anticancer drugs)
androgens and progestins (hormones)
Diethylstilbestrol (DES, a hormone)
mercury (present in some medications)
Accutane® (used to treat acne)

SUSPECTED TERATOGENS

lithium (a psychiatric drug)
Benzodiazepenes (tranquilizers)
certain oral contraceptives
amphetamines (stimulants, often taken for weight control)
Cortisone (an antiinflammatory)
certain antihistamines

CLASTOGENS

propranolol (an antihypertensive drug)
thiazides (diuretic drugs)
chloramphenicol (an antibiotic)
tetracyclines (antibiotics)
meprobamate (a tranquilizer)
reserpine (antihypertensive)
erythromycin (an antibiotic)
streptomycin (an antibiotic)

Over-the-Counter Drugs

PROVEN HUMAN TERATOGENS

ethyl alcohol

SUSPECTED HUMAN TERATOGENS

None

CLASTOGENS

aspirin
tobacco
caffeine
certain antihistamines
vitamins A, D, and K in excess

Under-the-Counter Drugs

CLASTOGENS

every one of them, from acid to grass

Common Medications That Are Probably Safe

penicillin and certain derivatives
acetaminophen
mild narcotics, such as codeine taken *occasionally* for pain

These lists are not complete, but they are close to being so. Nonetheless, in the over-the-counter field alone, there are close to a half-million products available, and it is difficult if not impossible to keep up with all of them.

Medical Complications of Pregnancy

The course of pregnancy is altered by coexistant diseases or problems that tend to complicate both the existing disease itself and the newly acquired pregnancy. We have already seen some of this in discussing high-risk obstetrics. There are a number of reasons for this expanding area of obstetrics. One is the increasing frequency of pregnancy in the older maternal population. Another is better medical control of many disorders that in the past ruled out pregnancy, made it difficult to achieve or impossible to consummate. A good example of what I am talking about is the relatively common medical condition known as diabetes. We will use this particular medical problem as an illustration. So listen.

Before insulin was discovered and became generally available, diabetes and pregnancy were almost incompatible. Diabetic women generally didn't live long enough to conceive, and if they did get pregnant, the combination was uniformly lethal to both mother and baby. Nowadays, thank goodness, pregnant diabetics, with help, can share the same happy and successful outcome as their unburdened peers. With help.

The effects of diabetes on pregnancy can be:

• abortion
• prematurity and postmaturity
• stillbirth
• congenital malformations
• large infants
• immature and sick infants
• hypertension of pregnancy
• and more

The effects of pregnancy on diabetes are:

• Marked changes in insulin requirements. Insulin needs may

decrease in early pregnancy but generally increase and fluctuate sharply in later pregnancy.

- Increased incidence of metabolic imbalance and tendency to develop acidosis. This dangerous metabolic change can develop silently and rapidly, particularly in late pregnancy.
- Increased dietary needs to nourish the developing pregnancy.

As you can see, all these conditions have a profound effect upon each other and require delicate and exquisite control. The management of a diabetic pregnancy usually, but not always, involves:

- Early hospital admission, for control and evaluation of the diabetes and the pregnancy and to establish rapport between the physician, the patient, nutritionists, and all others involved in this elaborate process.
- Meticulous control of the diet, which often involves a change in dietary habits and the initiation of frequent multiple feedings. The principle here is to prevent hyperglycemia (excess blood sugar), which is the most critically damaging effect diabetes can have on pregnancy.
- Insulin adjustment and constant readjustment. Today, with modern blood monitoring devices, most cooperative diabetics can assess their own blood sugar levels and adjust their diet and insulin dosages accordingly.
- Close monitoring of fetal activity and growth. This involves the use of nonstress and stress testing as well as biophysical profiles and amniocentesis (see Appendix).
- Close observation in late pregnancy for evidence of fetal lung maturity, and delivery at the optimal time, whenever that may be.
- Special management of "neglectors." Many problems with diabetic patients during pregnancy involve those who fail to follow instructions and advice. Such unfortunate mothers require special help and assistance for themselves and their babies.

Incidentally, the condition known as gestational diabetes occurs in expectant mothers who are potential diabetics and whose physiology will eventually yield to overt clinical diabetes. The metabolic and endocrine stress of pregnancy often produces a condition identical to diabetes and thus a pregnancy complicated with the same disorders as clinical diabetes. These patients require the same medical care as an actual diabetic.

This example represents a very brief encounter with a major medical disorder complicating pregnancy. There are many variations and substitutions among the procedures I have described that may alter the treatment that a pregnant diabetic will receive from her physician. Again, as always, the doctor's care is more intimate and personal—and important—than anything that might be revealed in this section.

This is only one example of the medical disorders that complicate pregnancy and vice versa. So while we are at it, let's just list some of the common as well as some of the bizarre medical problems in which pregnancy can exist successfully but that have this two-way impact on each other:

- problems in the gastrointestinal system
  malnutrition
  liver problems such as cirrhosis and hepatitis
  intestinal surgery, previous intestinal surgery such as bypass
    and stomach stapling procedures and large surgical re-
    sections for tumors
  crohn's disease (ulcerative colitis)
- problems in the renal system
  chronic infections (pyelitis)
  renal damage (nephritis and nephrosis)
  renal transplants
  renal dialysis
- problems in the cardiovascular system
  anemias of various types
  heart disease such as congenital or rheumatic heart disorders,

ischemic heart disease (angina and/or infarctions)
previous heart surgery for congenital or rheumatic heart
disease, or valve replacement and coronary artery bypass
procedures
hypertension and stroke
- problems in the endocrine system
diabetes
thyroid disorders
pituitary and adrenal gland disorders
- problems in the pulmonary system
asthma, emphysema, and pulmonary infections
previous surgery to lungs (lobectomy or pneumonectomy)
- problems of systemic infection
Torch Syndrome
AIDS
- problems in the central nervous system
epilepsy
migraine
multiple sclerosis
cerebral palsy
- cancer—mothers who have arrested cancers of various body
organs and systems

These various disorders are but a small sampling of the
medical problems that may complicate pregnancy. There are
many others, and they all serve as a great challenge to modern
obstetrical management.

Fascinating Facts

▷ In most ancient cultures the management of the umbilical
cord following delivery was handled in a very specific way.
In general, the cord was cut after the placenta was completely
delivered, but sometimes it was cut beforehand. Usually
separation was achieved at some distance from the baby, in

order that bleeding would not take place. Instead of being cut with a sharp instrument, it was generally chewed or ground apart with stones. Sometimes heat was used to separate it, and sometimes it was simply torn by the hands. It really didn't make much difference, since the placental circulation and, therefore, circulation through the cord ceases at the moment of a newborn child's first respiration.

▷ In ancient Arabic cultures, pieces of raw salt were put into the mother's vagina after she delivered. The purpose of this was to make the vagina shrivel enough so it would be tight in subsequent sexual encounters. The complications from this practice can be unbelievable. It is still carried out in some nomadic cultures today.

DIARY

My Fourth Month

Problems _____

Medications _____

_____

_____

Baby moved? When? _____

What's going on in the world? _____

_____

_____

What's going on in my life? _____

_____

_____

My thoughts and feelings _____

_____

_____

Doctor's Appointment _____

Questions To Ask

_____

_____

_____

_____

CHAPTER FIVE

MY FIFTH
LUNAR MONTH

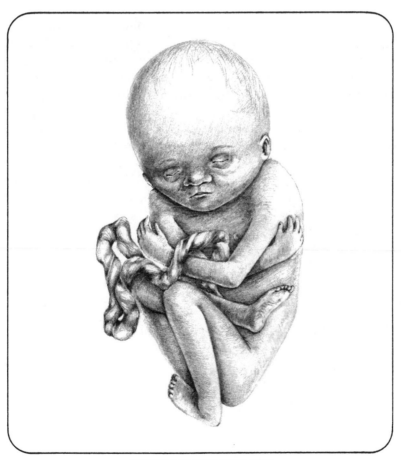

FIFTH LUNAR MONTH

The sixteenth to the twentieth weeks comprise the fifth lunar month of your pregnancy, and between your belly button and the bottom of your abdomen you have your own personal mountain, which, unlike Muhammad's, moves—in fact, it moves all the time. By now your child weighs ten ounces (300 grams) and is 7.2 inches (18 centimeters) long. It should be easy for your doctor to pick up the fetal heartbeat with an ordinary stethoscope, and it can be picked up very readily and most clearly for both of you to hear with the ultrasound monitor. This is a reassuring and enjoyable encounter indeed. There should be very little doubt in your mind about what is going on inside you, and since you are feeling regular movement, you know the heart must be beating whether you get to hear it or not. I'm sure there is no doubt in your mind that you are growing. Keep moving!

Immunization During Pregnancy

Sometimes vaccination dilemmas come up in pregnancy. Here is a summary of the known immunization facts.

Four types of immunizing agents are used in the United States.

- toxoids, which are chemically altered poisons secreted by bacteria

- killed bacterial and viral vaccines, which still retain their ability to produce immunity
- live virus vaccines, which have been altered so that they do not cause serious clinical illness but still produce immunity
- immune globulin preparations, a protein fraction of human plasma that can induce transient, passive antibody protection in the recipient

Women of childbearing age in this country usually are already immune to measles, mumps, rubella (German measles), tetanus, and diphtheria. Most women born prior to 1957 are considered immune to measles, mumps, and German measles because they most likely were infected with the disease. Those born after 1957 have probably been vaccinated; in fact, most everyone should now have been vaccinated against rubella. Immunity to rubella can be documented by a simple blood test. As far as diphtheria and tetanus are concerned, almost everyone has now universally been vaccinated, although booster doses are required every ten years for diphtheria and tetanus to keep the immune levels high.

As a general rule, vaccination with any immunizing agent during pregnancy should be limited to a few very clearly defined situations. Preferably, of course, all routine vaccinations have been carried out prior to pregnancy. This is not always the case and, further, some unusual exposures may take place. Each situation must be assessed in terms of the following:

- Risk of exposure. Pregnant women should avoid areas where certain infectious disorders are epidemic or endemic. As an example, avoid travel to areas where the plague or yellow fever exists—and there are areas of the United States where plague now exists. As another example, if you are a teacher, stay home when epidemics of rubella, flu, or chickenpox are active in your school.
- Risks from disease. When a pregnant woman is susceptible

and, further, is at risk of exposure to an infectious disorder, then the particular mortality and morbidity risks of the disease for her and her fetus must be assessed carefully by her doctors. Some infectious disorders are known to produce greater harm during pregnancy than at other times; rubella is a good example of this.

• Risk from immunizing agents. We have to further consider what risk the actual immunizing agents themselves might have upon the expectant mother, her health, and that of her fetus. Not much is known about the effect of most vaccines on pregnancy. One, however, that has been studied in great detail is rubella and its vaccine, and vaccination with this agent is definitely not recommended during pregnancy. On the other hand, diphtheria and tetanus vaccinations are apparently safe at this time.

These factors must all be weighed in making the decision of whether it is necessary or advisable to vaccinate during pregnancy, and all involved need to participate in this decision-making process.

Here follows a list of most of the immunizing agents used and their status for use during pregnancy.

Immunizing Agent	Indications for Immunization During Pregnancy
LIVE VIRUS VACCINES	
Measles	Contraindicated (see immune globulins)
Mumps	Contraindicated
Poliomyelitis	Not routinely recommended for adults in U.S., except persons at increased risk of exposure
Rubella	Contraindicated
Yellow fever	Contraindicated except if exposure is unavoidable

132

Immunizing Agent	Indications for Immunization During Pregnancy
INACTIVATED VIRUS VACCINES	
Influenza	Usually recommended only for patients with serious underlying diseases; public health authorities to be consulted for current recommendation
Rabies	Unknown
INACTIVATED BACTERIAL VACCINES	
Cholera	Unknown
Meningococcus	No data available on use during pregnancy
Plague	None reported
Pneumococcus	No data available on use during pregnancy
Typhoid	None confirmed
TOXOIDS	
Tetanus-diphtheria	Lack of primary series, or no booster within past 10 years
IMMUNE GLOBULINS: HYPERIMMUNE	
Hepatitis B	Postexposure prophylaxis
Rabies	Postexposure prophylaxis
Tetanus	Postexposure prophylaxis
Varicella	Not routinely indicated for healthy pregnant women exposed to varicella
IMMUNE GLOBULINS: POOLED	
Hepatitis A	Postexposure prophylaxis
Measles	Postexposure prophylaxis

Source: American College of Obstetricians and Gynecologists, "Immunization During Pregnancy," *ACOG Technical Bulletin,* Washington, D.C., no. 64, May 1982.

133

Traveling

By Air

Like most other activities during normal pregnancies, traveling offers few hazards. Flying is actually the safest way to travel, as long as the airlines will accept you. Although most airlines don't now require it, a few will still request a letter from your physician stating your air worthiness if you are in the last month.

Air travel is more comfortable and much faster than ground travel, and if something does happen stewardesses make better midwives than do service station attendants! Modern pressurized cabins offer no problems; there is no risk of ozone or radiation effect, and the greatest danger would probably be from passengers who smoke in these confined quarters. In this regard it seems entirely possible that smoking will shortly be banned on most short domestic flights. For further information on air travel, write to the Airtransport Association of America, 1709 New York Avenue, N. W., Washington, D. C. 20006.

By Car

If you travel by automobile you should observe the following rules:

- Travel no longer than eight hours a day.
- Stop frequently. Get out, walk around and stretch your limbs, and test all the local facilities.
- Carry some vitamin B_6 tablets with you in case you become carsick.

134

- Always fasten your safety belt, no matter how short the ride. Be sure that the lap belt is below the baby and riding on your thighs and that the shoulder harness gives you at least three inches of freedom in the upper chest area. The benefit to you and baby far outweigh any risks of compression or being trapped in the car. If you are driving the car yourself and are not buckled in, the steering wheel can represent a formidable weapon to both of you. Always buckle up.
- Do not make long trips without checking with your doctor first. There are certain times during your pregnancy when it might be unwise for you to be far from home base. Try to avoid travel during the first three months; although traveling itself does not induce a miscarriage, the roadside is no place to have one. Further, traveling during the last month should be avoided because labor may be imminent.

There is nothing worse than long-distance automobile traveling when you are low on gas, high on bladder pressure, tired, hungry, and thirsty, and it is often difficult to find a place to stop that offers all the facilities you need. There is a company that will send you, at a nominal charge, the names of some five hundred all-day, all-night auto-truck stops in the United States. These facilities are noted for gas and oil and bathrooms, but they also offer places to sleep, laundries, barbershops, post offices, banks, shopping centers, and the like. Such information might be of real value to you on a long trip. Write to the National Association of Truck Stop Operators, P.O. Box 1285, Alexandria, Virginia 22313; or call them at (703) 549-2100.

Unless there is something very abnormal with your pregnancy, you may travel within a thirty- to forty-mile radius of home at any time.

International Travel

If you plan to travel outside the United States, particularly in a foreign country where there may be a language barrier, there is an international medical agency that can give you a list of English-speaking physicians almost anywhere in the world. If you wish more information about this society or want their catalogue, write to the International Association for Medical Assistance to Travelers, Empire State Building, 350 Fifth Avenue, New York, New York 10001.

On a long trip, jet lag increases your fatigue, so be sure to take it easy the first 24 to 48 hours after your arrival. This fatigue is even more evident if you are flying to a place of higher altitude than your home. Mountain air sickness is a very common complaint, and there is some evidence that *some* unhealthy fetal conditions may occur if you fly to a higher altitude and try to go skiing the same day or even the next day. You should gradually acclimatize yourself, as I have noted, over at least a two-day period, before attempting any strenuous activity at higher altitudes during pregnancy. (This advice is just as good if you're not pregnant.)

Most countries no longer require vaccinations to enter or leave, but should you be headed for an exotic foreign land where diseases like cholera, smallpox, or plague may still exist, better check first—and read the section on immunization beginning on page 130.

In case you have been worried about the X-ray machines used at airport security areas, they do not yield a sufficient amount of radiation to affect your pregnancy.

If you are susceptible to diarrhea and are traveling abroad, remember that roughly half the Americans traveling outside the United States today get diarrhea. In order to minimize this, drink bottled water only. Avoid iced drinks, uncooked foods, and partially cooked meats. Peel all fruits and wash all vegetables.

Should you get diarrhea, take Pepto-Bismol®, which you should bring with you, and drink fruit juices, ginger ale, or other carbonated beverages; try adding some salt to them. Gatorade®, if available, is of great value in replacing fluids and electrolytes lost by diarrhea.

Accidents

Automobile Accidents

At least 7 percent of all pregnant women are involved in some sort of accident, and that doesn't include the original one. Automobile accidents, of course, head the list. Even in a minor accident you may not remember very much about the moment of impact, and so you may not be certain whether or not you received an abdominal blow. If you are able to, be sure to check at once by feeling around your tummy to see if there is any area of tenderness. Further, check for bruising. Also, as soon as you have a chance, try to determine if there has been any change in your vaginal secretion, and look in particular for the presence of blood or water. If there is the least doubt in your mind, go to a hospital and be examined, and be sure to get a fetal heart check. You may want to repeat the monitor check the next day in your doctor's office. Unless it is unavoidable, don't take any medication for pain or for anything unless your personal obstetrician or doctor orders it. In a major accident, if you are conscious, tell someone that you are pregnant, how far along you are in the pregnancy, and what your blood type happens to be.

Home Falls

Landing on your back or your side, if you fall, generally cushions the blow for the baby. But if the fall should be severe and sudden, it may indirectly produce damage to the baby. So if you fall, you must watch for abdominal pain, vaginal bleeding or fluid, and the amount of baby activity that is going on if the baby has already been moving. If you fall on or get hit on your abdomen, again look for pain or bleeding and the amount of baby activity. Call your doctor or go to a hospital and have them listen with the fetal heart monitor if you are in doubt. Sometimes after you have had a spill or a fright of some sort, your baby becomes very active. After all, baby is in there in the dark, standing on its head, unable to see or hear what's going on. No wonder it jumps around when you have a violent reaction to something!

Thermal Burns, Electric Shocks, and Lightning

Severe thermal burns usually do not affect the baby. Electric shocks can, depending upon where the current comes in and where it goes out. Again, look for these three cardinal signs: pain, vaginal bleeding, and loss of sensation of baby movement. Get a fetal-monitor check if necessary. Let your doctor know.

Even supposing we find out the very worst—that your baby has been lost even though you're okay—there is nothing that can now be done to change what has happened. We must accept it—and, moreover, it's important that we know. An infant no longer alive cannot be left inside you very long. However, on the brighter side, what a blessing it is after such injury to find out that your baby is alive and fine—and that's almost always the case!

Vaginal Bleeding

Vaginal bleeding anytime during pregnancy must be considered an abnormal sign (although it may not be) and should be reported to your doctor immediately. Often it signifies no great danger, but its importance should be evaluated by your doctor and no one else. As we have seen, bleeding in early pregnancy is a common sign of threatened or impending miscarriage. Now that you are further along, there are many other things that may cause vaginal bleeding, among them such minor conditions as infections of the vagina or the cervix and varicose veins in this area. Occasionally a small amount of spotting may be noted after sexual relations. This generally is due to irritation of the vagina and the cervix, but still, let your doctor know.

The most dangerous type of bleeding that can occur now is from the site of the placenta. Such bleeding usually signifies that part of the placenta has separated from the uterine wall; it may or may not be accompanied by pain. Whatever the other symptoms, you should call your doctor at once whenever vaginal bleeding appears.

Sometimes labor is initiated by the discharge of a plug of mucus from the cervix, which many times is stained with blood. This discharge is called show and is not a cause for worry. Labor may start within a few moments after the appearance of show, but it may not begin for several days. There is no need to call your doctor when show appears unless it is accompanied by other signs of labor, such as regular cramps, or unless the membranes rupture. These signs are dealt with farther along in the book.

Your Skin

Your skin undergoes many changes during pregnancy. For one, it is stretched like a drumhead. You can attest to that! For another, it is subject to the influence of hormones produced and secreted throughout pregnancy. With these two powerful inside factors, stretch and hormones, aided and abetted by the inroads of the atmosphere and any personal pollutants you may habitually apply in the name of beauty, your skin is likely to feel like the cover of a used weather balloon—and it may not look much better. On the other hand, there are women who have had skin problems all their lives who find, to their joy, that everything on the surface clears up during pregnancy so that their skin becomes shimmering, healthy, and more attractive than it has ever been. This is the "bloom of pregnancy" and is wonderful to behold.

Acne

The hormone changes that we mentioned may have adverse effects on the skin in early pregnancy and thus bring about changes on the face and neck that resemble acne. These lesions generally clear up as time goes on and should be managed by keeping your skin very clean, using a medicated soap and little makeup. The status of soaps that contain hexachlorophene is at this moment unclear. You can only consult your doctor.

Chloasma

Some women experience chloasma, a mottled darkening of the facial skin that usually becomes heaviest on the forehead, the bridge of the nose, and the cheeks below the eyes. This darkness usually disappears sometime after delivery, but it may be a source of mixed emotions during pregnancy. Cover it up—but gently—with something nice. Similar skin darkening may occur around the nipples and certain other body areas, but again, lightens after delivery. Avoid direct sunlight if you have chloasma.

Striae

One of the most distressing of the skin changes that may appear is a series of reddish lines on the abdomen, flanks, and breasts. These striae are more likely to occur in women with delicate skin. They represent the separation of deeper layers of the skin itself, allowing the reddish blood vessels and tissue underneath to show through. Some months after delivery, the redness vanishes and the lines become silvery white and much less noticeable. However, it is not likely that they will ever completely disappear. Little can be done to prevent striae from occurring, but it may help to do the following:

- Wear garments that provide good support for the breasts and the abdomen during pregnancy.
- Maintain a moderate weight gain.
- Massage the breasts and the abdomen daily with a good skin cream containing lanolin.

Red Dots

Very often little red dots appear on the neck and arms during pregnancy and increase in size irregularly as time does on. They are not very noticeable—except to the bearer—are harmless, and disappear after your baby is born.

Superficial Veins

All the superficial veins under the skin, under the influence of certain hormones, dilate while you are pregnant. These dilated vessels produce a variety of noticeable effects. The larger veins of the arms and hands, legs and feet become distended. Those of the lower extremities tend to stand out even more because of the increasing pressure of the growing pregnancy. Further, it is not unusual to notice a mottling effect on the lower extremities and the palms of the hands. There is nothing abnormal whatsoever about these changes, and they are only temporary. The treatment of abnormal varicose veins is discussed later on.

Rashes

There are several skin rashes that are liable to bother you.

- Iron supplements may produce a small pinpoint rash over your chest, abdomen, and back. Stop your vitamin-mineral supplement for a week (if your doctor approves). The rash should go away, proving the point, and your doctor will prescribe a different kind of iron.

- Pruritus of pregnancy. This is simply an itchy sensation all over, generally with no rash. No one knows the cause, but nothing serious comes of it—unless your fingernails are too sharp. Bathe daily in tepid water to which you have added a moisturizing lotion. After toweling, apply a lanolin cream; do so again at bedtime. If your itch seems unbearable, your doctor may prescribe a cortisone-based cream. Or he may rightly be opposed to it.
- Herpes of pregnancy. This skin disorder is totally related to pregnancy, and the cause is unknown. It usually begins toward mid-pregnancy, but it may start after delivery. You are covered with an itchy eruption, mainly on your arms, abdomen, upper chest, back, and thighs. (What's left?) This particular rash must be diagnosed and treated by your doctor or a skin specialist. Although rarely it *might* endanger your pregnancy, it is not closely related to the herpes virus that is so much in the news of late.
- You may have allergic rashes as a reaction to anything during pregnancy, just as at any other time. Thus, strawberries, tomatoes, nylon, pollen, jewelry, makeup—anything can give you "contact dermatitis." Watch what you put on—and put in.

Twins—and Others

Once you have found out for sure that you are pregnant, know when to expect delivery, and are aware that the sex cannot in any simple fashion be determined, your next question may well be, "Could I be carrying twins? Or triplets? Or . . . more?"

Well, you certainly could, particularly if you are over thirty and have several children already, if twinning is in your family history, and if your uterus has some abnormal shape. Your chances under such a combination of circumstances would be about one in twenty.

Ordinarily, you have about a one in eighty chance (slightly greater if you are black) of twinning, about one in eighty × eighty of having triplets, one in eighty × eighty × eighty for quadruplets, and so on. These are rough projections, and many things can affect them. A recent medical advance, for instance, that has altered this mathematical formulation is the advent of fertility drugs. Such drugs induce ovulation and, in large doses or in supersensitive individuals, may induce multiple ovulation and thus multiple fertilizations.

The rate of twinning varies throughout the world from very high—40 per thousand in Nigeria—to low—6.4 per thousand in the Orient. The rate of identical twinning is constant worldwide; it is the rate of fraternal twinning that alters these figures.

Here are some more facts about multiple pregnancies.

- Monozygotic twins are identical. They come from the initial split of one egg. Inheritance, maternal age, and number of previous children have no influence on identical twinning and, as noted, the rate is universally unchanged.
- Dizygotic (two-egg) or fraternal twins are definitely more common in older women with previous children and a family history of twins. Incidentally, twins do not skip a generation.
- *Superfetation* produces twins in an unusual way. It is based on the development of a second fertilized egg within a uterus that already contains a developing pregnancy fertilized in the previous cycle. Thus, the twins are different ages. *Superfecundation*, even more unusual, results when two or more eggs from the same cycle are fertilized by sperm from two different episodes of intercourse, either by the same or by a different male.
- As noted, malformation of the uterus (a double uterus, for example) seems to predispose toward twins.
- How to tell if twins are identical or fraternal:

If they are of different sexes, they are obviously fraternal. If the twins are in one sac, they must be identical.

If their sacs are separated by four layers of tissue (visible only under a microscope), the twins are fraternal. If only two layers separate them, they are identical.

One placenta (afterbirth) means identical twins, but two placentas or even co-joined placentas can occur in either type of twins.

In difficult differentiations, blood typing, fingerprints, and even chromosome analysis may be used to make the determination.

• Triplets and quadruplets may come from one egg, but this is unusual. More often several eggs are involved. The famous Dionne quintuplets, for instance, came from three eggs.

• Multiple births are generally born prematurely—three weeks early for twins, on the average—and of course then are smaller, not only because they are born early but because there is less room inside. Twins weigh about the same as singleton pregnancies up until about the twentieth week of gestation and thereafter gain at a consistently slower rate. Twins born in a first pregnancy are likely to be smaller than those in a later pregnancy. Identical twins tend to be smaller and to weigh about the same. They also, unfortunately, tend to have more deformities because the single egg may not split evenly or completely. The difference in weight may be much greater in fraternal twins, and certainly, if they are the result of superfetation, there may be a considerable difference. Also, one rascal may even steal nourishment from the placenta of its wombmate, and the weight difference here may be tremendous.

• Plural pregnancies and deliveries are subject to many more complications, such as anemia, hydramnios (excess amniotic fluid), hypertension of pregnancy, edema, difficult and premature labor, and delivery with abnormal presentation.

- Twins are generally but not always diagnosed before delivery. The doctor has a high incidence of suspicion when there is rapid weight gain and a rapid increase in uterus size, with many small parts to feel. Ultrasound examination reveals with almost 100 percent accuracy whether twins are present. Occasionally they are not detected because what appears to be a second fetal sac in early pregnancy may be either a false sac or a second embryo that reabsorbs (see Ultrasound in the Appendix). It may be that many pregnancies start out as twins and end up as singletons; only further ultrasound research will establish this. Ultrasound occasionally overlooks one baby of triplets or quadruplets, but it is, by and large, exceedingly accurate.

If you are expecting more than one child, it is important that you spend a fair part of the last third of your pregnancy at rest. You should be up only to take care of basic functions. You may be bothered by boredom, insomnia, swelling, and pressure, but bed rest is essential. Bed rest apparently does not hold back the onset of premature labor, but it helps prevent hypertension of pregnancy, a common complication with twins, and it does increase fetal nourishment and, therefore, fetal weight at the time of birth. This is all very important. While you are in bed, keep body muscle toned as much as you can by isometric exercise, but *no bearing down.* The management of labor and delivery of multiple births should generally be in a class II or class III obstetrical unit (see the discussion of Perinatal Centers in the Appendix, pp. 290–291). It can become a very complicated procedure, and the incidence of cesarean section is somewhat greater for twin deliveries than for singletons.

Backache and Posture

Perhaps one of the most significant differences between people and animals is our ability to walk erect, but, alas, our erect posture has led to that exclusively human disorder, the aching sacroiliac. The sacroiliac joint is your means of connecting two very important parts of you to each other—your top to your bottom—and thus this area is a common source of considerable discomfort when abused.

There are many ways of putting stress and strain and, eventually, damage into the sacroiliac joint. Pregnancy is one of them. Your growing baby acts like a weight and pulls you forward. To compensate for this, you lean farther back and increase the strain and the shearing effect on your sacroiliac area. If your partner can't understand how this happens, ask him to hang his bowling ball on his belt buckle!

After delivery, backache sometimes persists for long periods of time and may eventually develop into a chronic low back strain unless corrective postural exercises are done regularly or some supportive mechanism is worn. Various plans and devices can help combat the chronic sacroiliac strain:

- In early pregnancy try wearing an ordinary stretch girdle until it is no longer comfortable. Then a corsetiere, employed by a surgical supply house, can fit you with a maternity girdle that will give you excellent support for the remaining months of pregnancy. Although these girdles are much lighter in weight than the older variety, they actually are pretty restrictive and, in the summertime, very hot. Unless your back is extremely painful, it's probably better to avoid any kind of girdle, since these devices tend to do the work your muscles should be doing in the first place.
- Do postural exercises. Instruction booklets are generally available at your doctor's office.
- During periods of rest and upon retiring at night, sleep on your side, curled up as much as you can. This helps relieve the sacroiliac strain.
- Try local heat and massage, which are great temporary aids.
- Get into flat-heeled shoes to reduce the sacroiliac strain and discomfort.

- If it's absolutely necessary, take medicine that reduces the spasm and inflammation around the sacroiliac joint, but only under your doctor's supervision.
- After delivery, exercise. Vigorous postural exercises are preferable to wearing a girdle. You will find that you are getting plenty of exercise after you arrive home from the hospital and may not be pleased that your doctor suggests a few more. Actually, however, most of the work you do doesn't help your back a bit; it probably tends to make your strained joints more strained. Your back is going to have to carry you a long way and for a long time, so be kind to it.
- If you have a really bad back and chronic disability, write to the National Back Foundation, 24 Donaghey Building, 701 Main, Little Rock, Arkansas 72201.

Teeth for Two

Pregnant women are often warned by friends and relatives that their teeth are going to fall out while they are pregnant. For every child a tooth is a folklore saying that has survived from antiquity, and it drives dentists to the wall. Perhaps there is an element of truth in it, but if there is, research has failed to prove it. Calcium deposited in the teeth is ordinarily not available again to the circulation. So no matter how badly calcium is needed elsewhere, even for the bones and teeth of a developing infant, it generally cannot be reabsorbed from an expectant mother's teeth. Enamel is permanent; therefore, most cavities that occur during pregnancies are coincidental to and not caused by enamel loss. Moreover, if you faithfully take the prenatal vitamins your doctor prescribed, there is only a slight possibility of a calcium deficiency developing during your pregnancy. (Contrary to popular belief, milk may not be a good source of calcium during pregnancy. The calcium in milk is poorly absorbed by pregnant women. See page 200).

You should see your dentist early in pregnancy to be sure

your teeth are in good condition. Any dental work that is necessary may be done during pregnancy, but no gas anesthetics should be used. You may have any form of local anesthetic your dentist wishes to use. Elective extractions should be delayed.

An unusual swelling of the gums is seen during pregnancy. This is not due to any vitamin deficiency, as a rule, provided you are taking the vitamins ordered for you. The swelling is accompanied by a redness and tenderness of the gums that often produces bleeding on slight contact. It is due to the hormones that cause dilation of veins immediately under the gums, just as occurs in the skin. It disappears very rapidly after delivery.

Stuffy Nose and Ears

The same congestion of superficial veins that sometimes takes place in the gums is seen frequently in the mucous membranes of the nose and ear canals. When it occurs in the nasal passages, nosebleeds may be the result. As a rule, such bleeding doesn't last very long and the amount of blood lost is not great. Persistent, severe nosebleeds require the attention of a nose and throat specialist, since occasionally the dilated nasal veins rupture and so will have to be cauterized.

Congestion of veins in the ear canals produces a feeling that resembles rapid descent in an airplane or the stopped-up feeling you get in your ears after swimming. The unfortunate difference here is that the sensation is persistent. Various drugs and drops have been used, but with transient and poor results. Most often the condition, once it develops, persists until delivery and then is gone.

Fascinating Facts

▷ The incidence of twins is decreasing worldwide. No one knows why.

▷ In 70 percent of American twins, two eggs are involved. In Japan it is the exact reverse. No one knows why.

▷ A head-on collision between two cars each going only *ten* miles per hour will increase the weight of a newborn baby by 20 G forces. This would give the child an apparent and actual weight of 150 pounds! Few mothers can restrain that load. So after delivery, buckle up your baby, too.

▷ In a triplet pregnancy recently the first infant delivered at the twenty-third week. The pregnancy was maintained and the other two infants delivered at 37.5 weeks—ninety-nine days later!

DIARY

My Fifth Month

Problems _____

Medications _____

_____

_____

Rate of baby movement on a scale of 1–10 _____

What's going on in the world? _____

_____

_____

_____

What's going on in my life? _____

_____

_____

_____

My thoughts and feelings _____

_____

_____

_____

Doctor's appointment _____

Questions To Ask

_____

_____

_____

_____

_____

CHAPTER SIX

MY SIXTH
LUNAR MONTH

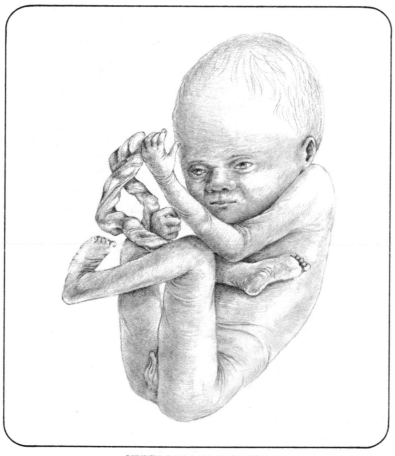

SIXTH LUNAR MONTH

You are now entering the sixth lunar month of your pregnancy—the twentieth to the twenty-fourth weeks. At the end of this period your baby weighs about a pound and a quarter, and its head is still by far the largest part of its body. Fat begins to be deposited under its skin, a very important factor in protecting it against temperature changes after birth. A child born at this time will attempt to breathe on its own and may survive in an intensive-care-nursery environment. A child weighing 14 ounces has survived. Incredible but true.

Baby moves inside you with a great deal more vigor. You find that it is somewhat more difficult to get about because of the increasing size of your lower abdomen, so you'd better be a little more careful about the way you move and the occasions on which you wear your heels.

Some companies used to suggest retirement about now. In a normal work environment, as we have already seen, this is no longer necessary or defensible. In some types of employment where there are physical hazards involved, it may be necessary to terminate work at an earlier time or to accept transfer to a less physically demanding type of work. Under such circumstances an employee's benefits and seniority will prevail in the future.

Intrauterine Growth Retardation (IUGR)

Although 8 percent of all babies delivered in the United States weigh under 2500 grams (5 lbs., 8 oz.) and are, therefore, premature by definition, they are not premature by actual dates. They are simply small for their gestational age and are suffering from intrauterine growth retardation (IUGR). Further, of those infants born weighing more than 2500 grams and, therefore, not premature by definition, some 5 percent may also actually be growth retarded.

There are two general categories of IUGR. The first is symmetrical, in which the whole body is reduced equally in size. The second is asymmetrical, in which the body is generally reduced to a greater degree than is the head. Symmetrical growth reduction is usually associated with an inherited fetal condition that is genetic in nature but may also be due to an injury sustained by the infant early in pregnancy, most likely from a systemic infection such as rubella or cytomegalovirus (see *Torch* Syndrome in chapter 4).

Asymmetrical growth retardation in the fetus is a complication of cardiovascular disease such as high blood pressure; of very old and very young mothers; of substance abuse such as cigarettes, drugs, or alcohol; of chronic maternal lung disease; severe anemia; and certain less common maternal conditions. The environment also apparently plays a role, since small babies are found at higher altitudes and in areas where expectant mothers are exposed to toxic substances (the Love Canal, for instance). Finally, multiple pregnancy will produce IUGR, as will certain disorders of the placenta.

If a doctor is suspicious that IUGR may take place, close observation of fetal growth is very important. When maternal abdominal enlargement fails to keep up with the pregnancy dates, ultrasound study is indicated. Not only does ultrasound establish the diagnosis, it differentiates between the two types of IUGR and can further assess fetal health with a biophysical profile (see Appendix, pp. 283–284). Other diagnostic tools and procedures are used to detect and follow IUGR, but none is as reliable as ultrasound (see Appendix, pp. 281–284).

IUGR is managed by providing the infant with the best internal environment possible for the remainder of its time in the uterus. This includes extra maternal bed rest, adequate nutrition, cessation of substance abuse, and removal from any damaging environmental factors. Close observation of fetal well-being and regular testing for fetal stress and distress are important. The tests are explained in the Appendix (see pp. 286–288). It is, unfortunately, often necessary to empty the uterus early if evidence of reduced placental reserves or fetal distress is shown. In such cases labor must be watched very closely for increased fetal distress, so there is a higher incidence of delivery by cesarean section in cases of IUGR.

The long-term outcome for these babies depends upon the initiating factor, but generally, symmetrical growth retarded infants remain small as infants and children and also exhibit continued neurological abnormalities. On the other hand, asymmetrical retarded infants are more likely to catch up on their growth after birth, and they have fewer neurological abnormalities.

Hypertension of Pregnancy

This condition, also known as pregnancy-induced hypertension (PIH), has in the past contributed heavily to maternal and fetal mortality and disability. Although it is still a major problem and we still do not understand everything about it, modern medical management has greatly reduced the risks to both mother and baby.

What is it? PIH is a disorder limited almost exclusively to the last trimester of pregnancy. It generally strikes young women having their first baby as well as older women in any pregnancy;

women with preexisting high blood pressure, kidney disease, diabetes; and, in particular, women of low socioeconomic status who have chronic malnutrition. (Note, though, that many well-to-do women are also chronically malnourished—by choice.) PIH is characterized by a triad of symptoms, namely high blood pressure (hypertension), swelling of the tissues (edema), and albumin in the urine (proteinuria).

Why does it occur? The number of theories advanced is limitless. This tells you something about our knowledge. Yet all people who work with the disorder agree that it is strictly limited to pregnancy—to human pregnancy—and that almost always it is restricted to the third trimester. One of its major dangers is a reduction in blood flow (ischemia) to vital maternal organs, including the uterus. Thus the placenta feels the onslaught of ischemia and, in a reflex maneuver, puts out a substance to raise maternal blood pressure and, therefore, increase the pumping pressure of blood to it and to the fetus. Sadly, it doesn't work, and the abnormal condition is only worsened, as is the fetal blood supply. So the vicious cycle continues, putting the fetus in distress and jeopardy. Moreover, maternal damage from organ ischemia can be overwhelming and permanent. Thus when pregnancy is over, the placenta gone, and the disease abates and disappears, the mother may be left with high blood pressure, kidney disease, or other crippling problems.

At the onset PIH is generally mild; this is certainly the easiest time to institute treatment. Should the problem go unchecked, however, the high blood pressure, with failure of circulation through vital areas, makes treatment more difficult and vastly increases the risk of convulsions. This end point in the march of PIH is critical and demands instant control followed by delivery no matter the stage of pregnancy or the maturity of the child. This hazardous convulsive climax in the progression of PIH was traditionally and probably still is called eclampsia. Obstetricians, indeed everyone, dread to see the convulsive state, which can generally be avoided by adequate care and adherance to instructions (compliance, remember?) given here and, most important, by your own doctor.

The clinical management of PIH, then, depends upon the state of the disease and the duration of pregnancy. If the onset takes place when the pregnancy is at maturity or closely approaching it, the treatment is to control the blood pressure, prevent convulsions, and deliver the infant by the safest possible method. Usually this involves induction of labor, but sometimes, for a variety of reasons, cesarean section may have to be performed.

If the disease occurs while the infant is still premature, and if it is severe and accompanied by evidence of jeopardy to the infant or by intrauterine growth retardation (IUGR), the treatment is still the same—namely, control the blood pressure, prevent convulsions, and initiate procedures to start labor. If PIH is mild and the infant is premature, then conservative management is possible. The most important step is *bed rest* in a lateral position. This is probably the single greatest factor in preventing deterioration of PIH, since pressure is taken off the major vessels and circulation to the uterus is vastly improved. Such patients have to be followed in the hospital or in the doctor's office with regular blood pressure readings, urine checks, certain blood chemistry determinations, and certainly with very close watch on the fetus. This involves stress testing, nonstress testing, or biophysical profiles (see Appendix, pp. 281–288). When maturity is reached or if the treatment fails, then delivery in the most expedient manner is mandatory, as we have already seen. Once convulsions have set in, rapid delivery becomes imperative.

It must be pointed out again that these are broad, general outlines of treatment, which have to be tailored individually to patients with specific problems, and the best local tailor is your own physician. As an example, although we have said immediate arrangements for delivery must be made when convulsions occur, it is sometimes necessary to alter and correct body functions, fluid balance, urine excretions, electrolyte imbalance, and so forth before adding the extra burden of labor and delivery. Again, *your own physician knows best.*

What can you do yourself to prevent PIH from endangering your pregnancy? The most important approach you can take in this regard is adequate nourishment before and during your pregnancy, restriction of your sodium intake during all of pregnancy, and adequate rest in a lateral position during the last trimester. In the unfortunate event that you should become involved with PIH, you must follow your doctor's advice closely. But remember, watch your diet, get adequate rest, and report promptly any abnormal tissue swelling, headaches, spots before your eyes, reduction in fetal activity, or other symptom or sign that appears abnormal to you.

Relaxin Symptoms

In every pregnancy a variable amount of a hormone substance called relaxin is secreted, probably by the anterior pituitary gland. This hormone substance has but one purpose, and that is to relax the ligaments around your pelvis and hips in order that they stretch more easily during labor and thus ease your baby's trip. An unfortunate side effect of this ligament relaxation, however, is a feeling of pelvic instability. You may feel as if your hips are going to come out of their sockets, particularly when you first get out of a chair or out of bed. This relaxation of the joints is responsible for the "crick" and "catches" in your hips (not your back) and for the pain you often feel in the bottom of your abdomen as the pubic bones begin to separate.

Little can be done to ward off this feeling, but, like so many other things we have spoken about, it will disappear as soon as you deliver. Promises, promises!

Varicose Veins

We have talked about pressure on rectal veins caused by the growing baby. This pressure can cause hemorrhoids. Pressure is also transmitted to blood vessels in the lower extremities, producing a tendency toward varicose (swollen) veins. These may become more of a problem with each pregnancy. Pressure increases as pregnancy progresses, and not only do the veins become swollen, but there is some risk of complications developing within them. For this and for cosmetic reasons, therefore, it is important to take care of such abnormal veins if they develop during your pregnancy. First of all, never wear constricting circular garters to hold your hose up, and never roll your hose. (I don't think anyone does that anymore, but if you do, don't.) Second, try to avoid standing for long periods of time without rest or without moving around. Third, in all cases in which the veins have become a problem, wear some form of supportive hose. Relatively inexpensive, indeed almost attractive, hose for pregnancy that gives adequate support in most cases can now be bought at most drug or department stores. If more help is needed, your doctor will order special supportive hose for you at a surgical supply house. They look like cigar wrappers—but they work!

Particular Problems of Young and Older Expectant Mothers

If you have been paying attention, you already know about such conditions as high-risk pregnancy, PIH, IUGR, the whole bit, and you are now properly depressed about all the things that can happen to you as you mosey down maternity trail. Well, let's continue the litany and check out the problems of young and older mothers.

Here are the most common problems that are presented by an adolescent pregnant woman:

- Incomplete body growth of the expectant mother herself. Therefore, she is competing with her baby for nutrients, and both suffer.
- More low-birth-weight-for-date babies (IUGR).
- More premature babies.
- Increased cephalo-pelvic disproportion (between baby's head and mother's pelvis).
- Greater incidence of PIH.
- Greater incidence of cesarean section.
- Greater incidence of bad eating habits and anemia.
- Mother less likely to seek competent help early in pregnancy or to follow advice when sought.

And in the case of the more mature mother-to-be:

- Greater incidence of medical complications such as diabetes, hypertension, and renal disease.
- Greater incidence of congenital disorders in the newborn.
- Labor more likely to be ineffectual and require help.
- Cesarean section rate higher.
- Risks of the whole gamut of obstetrical complications in multiparous older mothers (women who have had many children).
- Possible permanent and irreversible effects in older women of the complications of prolonged smoking and other body abuse.

From the doctor's point of view, it's probably easier to take care of the older mothers-to-be. They seem to realize better what is at stake and to follow advice much more closely and do everything they can to protect their pregnancy.

In spite of reliable birth control and abortion on demand, there is still a very high proportion of unwanted pregnancy in our country, the vast majority of which occurs in teenage girls.

It is estimated that 1 girl in 10 becomes a mother before she graduates from high school—about 1,000,000 this year, of which some 600,000 will go on to deliver. Adolescent mothers are beset not only by the problems I have mentioned but also by a host of fundamental emotional problems derived from having to adapt to their new role as a mother before they have adapted to the role of a growing girl. As one of them put it, "One minute I was a running, ripping, hopping, jumping fourteen-year-old girl. Then I got pregnant." Going from age thirteen to twenty in nine months is a very long, hard jump. These youngsters are also confronted by the problem of very seldom having an understanding relationship with their parents, physician, or counselor. Such an unfortunate mother is many times advised to have an abortion when she doesn't want one, to have a baby when she doesn't want one, to marry when she doesn't want to, to not marry when she wants to, and to give up something or someone that she loves dearly. It is sometimes difficult for adults to remember that the desires of love and the sorrows of loss are felt just as greatly by youngsters as by adults. They are not forgotten any sooner or with any less trauma. They just occur at an earlier age.

Pregnant adolescents need a great deal of help, that is certain. It would take a separate chapter to outline their needs and a whole book to answer them. Here, however, are some suggestions:

- Search out an adult in the health-care field—your doctor, a nurse practitioner, a trained social worker—someone to whom you can relate and in whom you can confide and can bond with. You will be surprised how easy they are to find and how eager they are to help. Share your problems with them— they will give you the best help you can get.
- Eat carefully. Avoid junk food and salt. A recent study shows that 30 percent of all high school students tested had abnormally high blood cholesterol levels and that one in eight was

overweight. Don't jeopardize your growth and your baby's growth.

- If you smoke, quit. If you don't, don't start. Avoid alcohol and any drugs of any kind for any purposes.
- Take your vitamins and minerals as given to you.
- Continue to strengthen your relationship with your bonding person, and listen to the advice you get. That is the most important thing I call tell you.

Pets

Most American households harbor one or more pets. The emotional and physical benefits derived from the human-animal bond are well recognized, and the therapeutic value of the bond has been well established and documented. On the other hand, domestic animals that you have raised and loved can and do harbor conditions that may affect you during your pregnancy and, indeed, at any time.

The common household dog that provides a great deal of companionship and protection may also be host to a number of parasites that can infect the whole family. The most common of these offenders is the pinworm, which is not a serious infestation itself but is easily spread throughout a whole family. When this takes place everyone—human and canine—must be purged of the parasite. Under ordinary circumstances there is no problem in having the whole family take the necessary indicated medication. However, such medication should not be taken by a pregnant woman, particularly during the first trimester of her pregnancy. Thus, she will have to wait to rid herself of the scourge, meanwhile possibly reinfecting family members who have already been treated.

Dogs harbor a number of other organisms that can and are transmitted to humans. But the most serious of these is rabies, which presents a particular dilemma during pregnancy (see the discussion of immunization beginning on p. 130). It is important that you keep your dog's immunizations current for this and, of course, many other reasons.

Cats are another, more serious problem. Scratches and bites from household cats are a common occurrence. Moreover, cats are innate hunters and are likely to be exposed to anything infectious or toxic that has injured their prey. Rodents, which are a significant portion of their prey, can be infested with any number of deadly or crippling organisms. We have only to remember the plague-infested squirrels in Denver's city parks as a recent example of urban infestation. And, indeed, there was a very recent report of a child dying from the plague after allowing an infected pet cat to lick his face. Moreover, since cats lick their paws, and, therefore, their claws, these areas are frequently a source of infection, as are their bites. One particular bacteria that is a normal resident of the cat's mouth can produce fever and lymph gland enlargements, which are similar to symptoms of plague or tularemia. Finally, and of great importance during pregnancy, cats are a major source of human infection of toxoplasmosis, which has a devastating effect on pregnancy (see *Torch* Syndrome in chapter 4).

It may sound from all of this that I don't think much about cats; that is not true. I think about them a great deal, and I think they should be banished during pregnancy. If you keep a cat, at least an inside cat, avoid all close contact, licks, scratches— and avoid litter boxes. And avoid outside cats like the plague!

Although dogs and cats are the usual representatives of the animal world in our households, numerous other species may be found, including fish, birds, reptiles, and rodents. Since we usually have frequent intimate contact with these common inhabitants of our domestic environment, we must not overlook their attendant hazards.

As a general rule, do not make pets of or approach any wild animals or birds. They may harbor rabies, various viruses, bacterial infections, and fungus, and as we have noted, in the western United States, the plague. When all things are considered, your husband is probably your safest pet—but only by a slight margin!

Fascinating Facts

▷ At term, a healthy fetus can swallow 450 cc of amniotic fluid daily. This coincides with the amount of milk that a newborn infant can daily swallow the first few weeks after birth.

▷ Maternal smoking during pregnancy increases the risk of stillbirth or of infant death within a month after birth by 20–35 percent, and increases the risk of premature labor by 36–50 percent.

DIARY

My Sixth Month

Problems _____

Medications _____

_____

_____

Rate of baby movement on a scale of 1–10 _____

Natural childbirth classes _____

_____

_____

What's going on in the world? _____

_____

_____

_____

What's going on in my life? _____

_____

_____

_____

My thoughts and feelings _____

_____

_____

_____

Doctor's appointment _____

Questions To Ask

_____

_____

_____

CHAPTER SEVEN

MY SEVENTH
LUNAR MONTH

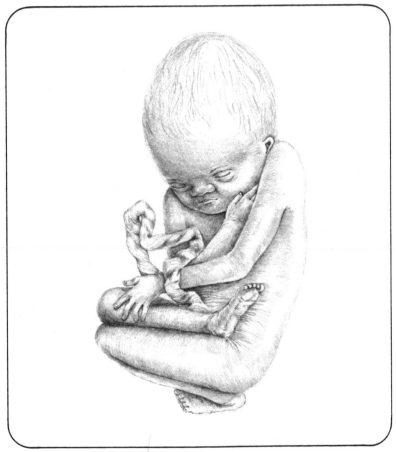

SEVENTH LUNAR MONTH

These are the twenty-fourth to twenty-eighth weeks of your pregnancy. There are still twenty-four hours in a day, but you feel like you're up twenty-eight. Your precious burden now weighs around two pounds. It is covered with a material called vernix caseosa, a white, cheesy, waxy substance that protects its skin much as grease protects ocean swimmers. If, by chance, labor begins and your baby is born at this age, it has a good chance to survive in an intensive-care nursery with an attendant neonatologist. It will breathe quite actively, move its limbs, and cry weakly.

It is often said that a child born at the end of the seventh month has a better chance of survival than one born at the end of the eighth month. This is absolutely incorrect! One of the most important things to remember is that in a normal pregnancy, every day a child remains in the uterus until full term increases its chances of survival.

As for your symptoms, while everyone else is freezing, you'll be fanning yourself. Lying flat in bed may make you short of breath, and you may notice your heart fluttering (palpitations) from time to time, whether you are resting or working. All these things are normal. Bless you.

Heartburn and Other Digestive Disturbances

Perhaps you thought when you finished early pregnancy that eating was forevermore going to be an endless and joyous indulgence, within the limits dictated by your scale and your pocketbook. You are now becoming aware that this is not so. In the first place, heartburn often becomes a regular companion. If you have never experienced heartburn before, it is a hot, irritating sensation in the lower chest, usually present after meals or before bedtime. It is worse if you have eaten fried or highly seasoned foods—which you are not supposed to be eating anyway, and you know it. Your partner can share this experience by swallowing a cigar.

Heartburn cannot be cured during pregnancy. It can, however, be temporarily relieved by the following:

• Avoid fried, greasy, or highly seasoned foods.
• Take frequent sips of (skim) milk or, better still, chew cracked ice.

Avoid any antacid preparations that contain sodium carbonate or sodium bicarbonate, and do not take baking soda or any similar preparation. If you need an antacid, have your doctor recommend one for you.

In late pregnancy, your stomach is pushed way up under your chest, thus often becoming congested and a very ineffective repository for food. Indigestion, nausea, and vomiting may result, particularly if you eat too much and too well. Therefore, it is important, as it was in early pregnancy, to avoid big meals and not to lie down after you eat.

A rare condition, diaphragmatic (epigastric, hiatus) hernia, produces severe, sometimes uncontrollable nausea and vomiting in late pregnancy and requires very special care. As with so much else, the hernia disappears with delivery.

Pressure Symptoms

By this time your friends have already given you blow-by-blow and push-by-push details about pressure symptoms in late pregnancy. Now you know what they were talking about and—for once—they were right. Just as the weight of the expanding uterus changes the position of the stomach and affects its ability to digest food, so the baby pushes against other abdominal organs and packs them up against your diaphragm. This pressure prevents the diaphragm from expanding adequately when you breathe, and thus you feel the shortness of breath that is so common in late pregnancy.

Sometime during the last month your baby may drop rather suddenly into your pelvis. This so-called lightening does not always occur before the onset of labor, but if it does, you will experience great relief in your upper abdomen and chest. You will be able to breathe more easily and eat more readily without digestive disturbances, and by and large you will feel a great deal more comfortable. On the other hand, your baby may descend more slowly into the pelvis over a period of weeks, and the upper abdominal relief may thus be less striking. At any rate, what is no longer up is down, and the pressure in your lower abdomen and pelvis increases, causing you seemingly ceaseless trips to and from the bathroom. Have faith and endure; relief is on the way!

Cesarean Section

The process of delivering a child by incision through the abdominal wall and the uterus has been known since prehistoric times, as indicated in early cave paintings in Africa. As recently as two hundred years ago a famous British obstetrician named Smellie had this to say about cesarean section in his textbook on obstetrics:

When a woman cannot be delivered by any of the methods hitherto prescribed and recommended in laborious and preternatural labors on account of narrowness or distortion of the pelvis into which it is sometimes impossible to introduce the hand—in such emergencies, if the woman is strong and of good habit of body, the cesarian operation is certainly advisable and ought to be performed because the mother and the child have no other chance to be saved. It is better to have recourse to an operation which *sometimes* succeeds than leave them both to inevitable death.

This was the state of cesarean operations at that time. It was mainly—almost exclusively—performed on women who were at the point of death or actually dead, with no hope of saving the mother, only of obtaining a live child. It had been thus since antiquity. When it was attempted on a living woman, she almost invariably died thereafter.

One hundred years later the results were not much better. A textbook written at that time reported that three-quarters of the living women on whom the operation was performed subsequently died.

Today, of course, cesarean sections are a relatively safe operation, and there are many hospitals in this country and elsewhere that have *never* experienced a maternal death from the cesarean procedure. All this is due to modern surgical techniques, anesthesia, antibiotics, and blood replacement, as well as, in broad terms, a healthier population and an increasing store of obstetrical wisdom and judgment. None of it is due to legislation, government interference, or activist groups. On the other hand, any one of these forces may and probably will reverse the magnificent trend now taking place.

The operation, as we have seen, was known to very early African cultures as well as to the Greeks, the Egyptians, and the Chinese at the height of their cultures; but again, the operation was probably resorted to only after the death of the mother. Pliny the Elder, the Roman naturalist, claimed in his writings that the renowned general Scipio, who defeated Hannibal, was the first thus brought into the world. But this is not so. However, the operation's name is derived from Roman culture. From being cut out of their mothers' wombs, such Roman individuals were first termed *caesons* and afterward *caesares*. To quote directly from the Latin source, *"Quia caeso matris utero in lucem prodiscunt."* This quote, which I can barely translate, says that a child should be removed from the uterus if its mother should die in late pregnancy. This law was known initially as the *lex regia* and continued under the rule of the caesars, thus acquiring the name *lex caesaria* and those delivered in this manner becoming known as *caesares*. Julius Caesar is said to have been brought into the world this way, but it is erroneous to state that the name Caesar was given to him on this account or that the operation was named for him.

Many reasons exist today for performing a cesarean section, the most common being a previous cesarean section. Though cesarean sections are almost always repeated in subsequent pregnancies, this is not any longer an absolute rule. Say, for instance, that toward the end of a normal pregnancy the membranes rupture, and as a result, the baby's umbilical cord prolapses or tumbles out of the uterus into the vagina. Under the right circumstances, a quick cesarean section will probably save the baby's life, provided it can be done before the umbilical cord is pinched off and the baby's oxygen supply thus terminated. Now, in this particular mother's next pregnancy, assuming that the same incident doesn't occur (and it is not likely to), will she need to be sectioned anyway? Not necessarily. Many factors enter into the decision regarding a possible vaginal delivery in her case. Much has been made of this change recently, both by the press and government, and indeed, some consensus rules have been established concerning the procedures to be followed in such circumstances. Probably the most important of these is that when normal labor is to be attempted and conducted upon a woman who has had a previous cesarean section, it must be so conducted in a hospital that is prepared to do an *immediate* cesarean section should an urgent complication arise, such as uterine rupture. Not many hospitals in the United States can qualify twenty-four hours a day for this particular exclusionary rule. Because of the unpredictable nature of obstetrics, even the best-staffed hospital may at one time have all its delivery and operating rooms full and busy, with more cases waiting to get in.

Other reasons for cesarean sections are disproportion between the mother's pelvis and the baby's head; abnormal presentation of the baby (such as breech position); hemorrhage from a separated placenta; certain medical conditions, such as diabetes, hypertension of pregnancy, and Rh disorders; multiple pregnancies with abnormal presentation of one or more infants; and many other more unusual problems. Practically none of these indications is absolute, and a great deal of judgment must be exercised in deciding whether to perform a section.

Although a great number of cesarean sections are performed before the onset of labor, it is safe in some instances to allow labor to proceed and to observe maternal and fetal conditions during labor, instituting the operation only if it seems wiser than allowing labor to progress and vaginal delivery to occur. It is almost never too late in labor to stop and do a cesarean section.

How many cesarean sections can safely be performed on one mother? Well, it used to be said that two was the maximum; after that the uterine scar became too weak and there was a possibility that it would rupture in a subsequent pregnancy. This danger has largely been eliminated by modern surgical techniques, and there is usually no reason to set a specific limit on the number of sections other than population and pocketbook.

The type of anesthesia used in sections varies with the conditions involved. From a review of the literature, it would appear that a spinal or epidural anesthetic (see Anesthesia and Analgesia, p. 235) is the most desirable form of pain relief, but this is not always so. There are times when such conduction anesthesia is absolutely contraindicated, and intravenous or inhalation anesthesia is to be preferred. This is a question of judgment involving you, your obstetrician, and the anesthesiologist. A review of all the factors involved is too complex to outline here. But your doctor and anesthesiologist should always discuss them with you and your partner should the situation arise.

There are two types of cesarean section. The classical operation is performed by making a vertical incision in the upper part of the uterus. It has the advantage of being very, very quick and avoiding the placenta, should it be lying very low and anterior in the uterus. It has the disadvantage of being more likely to form adhesions and being slightly more likely to rupture in future pregnancies. It is not usually performed today. The current standard cesarean section is a low cervical operation that constitutes a transverse incision in the very lowest part of the uterus. It takes somewhat longer to perform but generally heals much better, minimizes intraabdominal complications, and decreases the chance of future rupture. The only other type of cesarean section that may be used in modern obstetrics is the cesarean hysterectomy, in which case the uterus is removed following delivery. This would be done, for instance, if the mother had a compelling serious disease of the uterus that would require surgery in the near future, such as multiple tumors, noninvasive cervical cancer, or even certain problems that might arise during the cesarean section.

Many times when a patient is having difficulty in labor, her doctor is presented with this plea from an anguished family: "Why not go ahead and do a cesarean and get it over with?" Here again the answer cannot be given simply. There are many factors involved that have to be weighed and measured. By and large, delivery by the natural vaginal route is to be preferred, and a cesarean section does not always solve the problem with which we are faced. Indeed, sometimes it complicates and expands the problem at hand. The most important fact to keep before you is that you must have faith in your doctor and his or her associates and believe that their decision is based on the best interests of both you and your child. Fortunately, no obstetrician today is faced with the dreadful dilemma of sacrificing a mother for a child. This simply does not exist anymore. An unborn child is sometimes subjected to an increased risk in our decision making, but almost never a certain death.

Recovery following a cesarean section is generally rapid. There is some abdominal discomfort because, after all, surgery was performed. Generally speaking, however, the duration of the hospital stay is only slightly increased or not increased at all.

The cesarean-section "rate" in most accredited American hospitals varies between 10 to 20 percent of all deliveries. This rate is watched very closely by obstetricians who are responsible for staff doctor performance at the hospitals and also by a board of observers who tour the country, accrediting all American hospitals. Obstetricians are never checked or observed by any other groups, even when the hospital is religiously affiliated. If the cesarean-section rate is too high or too low or if there are maternal or fetal deaths that cannot be absolutely explained and accounted for, the obstetricians involved are in danger of losing their privileges to perform such operations and the hospitals are in danger of losing their all-important accreditation.

Heart Changes and Palpitations

Your heart is called upon to do a great deal of extra work during pregnancy. The volume of blood that it has to pump increases by 20 to 25 percent, and it becomes a great deal more difficult to circulate this blood because of the hemodynamics involved. For example, the growing baby exerts marked reverse pressure against the drainage of blood from your lower extremities. This is why expectant mothers who have heart disease

177

must be watched very closely as pregnancy progresses.

The normal heart can take the added stress without any serious limitations whatsoever. It is moved out of position by the rising diaphragm and winds up considerably left of center. This sometimes makes your heartbeat more readily felt, and since there are occasional episodes when your heart will beat much more rapidly (palpitations), the new experience may be somewhat frightening. In a normal heart these changes are never dangerous and soon stop if ignored. In the presence of heart disease, however, very special instructions are given during pregnancy, and these must be followed closely.

Leg Cramps

It is 4 A.M. and you have been to the bathroom ten times tonight, and even the Late Late Show is over. You are trying to catch a few moments of delicious sleep when zap!—it hits you. Your legs pull up in one tremendous cramp that throws you out of bed, or causes you to writhe and kick and grab at your legs until your husband is convinced that you are possessed. What's happening now?

What's happening is a tetanic contraction of your leg muscles due to a disturbance of calcium metabolism, brought about by—who knows what? But even though the disturbance is not completely understood, correction is relatively simple. First of all, eliminate milk from your diet. As we have already noted, milk in large amounts is not now considered important during pregnancy, particularly if your diet is otherwise adequate in protein and if you have been taking your vitamin-mineral supplements regularly. Milk is not necessarily a good source of calcium for pregnant women; in fact, it may prevent some calcium from getting into your system. Therefore, no milk. But be sure you are getting other adequate protein.

If that fails to stop your leg cramps, then double your prenatal vitamin-mineral supplement: take a pill morning and evening.

If your leg cramps do not disappear in a few days, you should consult your doctor for extra calcium pills. When the cramps do occur, get up and move around. Massage your leg or let your husband do it, or get into a tub of hot water.

Certain other muscular discomforts occur in late pregnancy, but these are generally due to the relaxation of ligaments and other supports of the pelvic bone.

Rh Blood Disorders

A great deal has been written about the importance and dangers of the Rh blood factor in association with pregnancy, but in reality very few babies are lost or damaged by the condition, and because of the new vaccine available, it has become even less of a problem.

Here's what it's all about. The Rh factor is a protein substance present in the blood of about 85 percent of all humans. They are therefore Rh positive. The remaining 15 percent, lacking the Rh factor, are therefore Rh negative. The Rh factor, like the color of the eyes, is inherited. It does nothing and goes nowhere. It is important only during blood transfusions and during pregnancy. When a blood transfusion is to be given, it is important that the Rh factors are matched. Actually, an Rh positive person can receive Rh negative blood without any difficulty or reaction, but the reverse is certainly not true.

In pregnancy, trouble may arise when the father is Rh positive and the mother Rh negative. The unborn child has an 85 percent chance of being Rh positive. During pregnancy and more likely during delivery, some Rh positive blood from the baby escapes into the circulation of its Rh negative mother. Since this blood contains a foreign protein substance, the mother begins to build up antibodies against it. (This is governed by the laws of immunity, in which a body tends to build antibodies against any foreign protein that appears within it—the basis for vaccinations and inoculations against diseases.) These antibodies are protective to their host—the mother. All would be fine, except that some of these antibodies can get back into the baby's circulation across the placenta and proceed to destroy the baby's blood cells, since they are antibodies, as noted, against such Rh positive cells.

Since it usually takes a pregnancy and delivery to initiate the process, there is almost never any difficulty with the Rh factor in the first pregnancy because *that* pregnancy is the sensitizing one. But in subsequent pregnancies, if preventive vaccine has not been given, the baby may be born anemic, jaundiced, or, worst of all, dead. However, there are now tests that can be performed on an Rh negative mother's blood (Coombs' test) as well as other procedures that can be done on the amniotic fluid during pregnancy to determine whether this sensitization is occurring. As an example of the amniotic fluid tests, a spectro-photometric analysis is commonly done. This procedure measures the optical density of amniotic fluid. The density becomes abnormal when blood pigment from the baby is present, and it is only present when the baby's blood is being destroyed by Rh disease.

In the event of significant sensitization as evidenced by blood or amniotic fluid studies, the uterus is emptied by an induction or cesarean section, unless, of course, the pregnancy is too immature. Under these circumstances we have developed a technique of transfusing the baby while it still lies within the uterus. This technique is rarely used today, however, because a vaccine is available which, given at the end of each pregnancy, counteracts the Rh antibody production in the mother and so protects her next child. Since the vaccine has become available, Rh disease of the newborn has become exceedingly rare, and it is hoped that such disorders will eventually be completely within our control. The vaccine is given during the first few days following birth, after special tests performed upon the mother and baby determine it is correct to do so. Rh negative vaccine is also given to Rh negative women who abort spontaneously or who have a therapeutic abortion or an ectopic pregnancy. Moreover, it is now becoming popular to give the vaccine to Rh negative women at about the twenty-eighth week of pregnancy, providing the Coombs' test is negative. This is an added protective factor for the mother and baby. Although the procedure has been used in other countries for some time, it has only recently been cleared by the Food and Drug Administration in this country to give to expectant mothers prior to full term and prior to delivery.

If you are Rh negative—and you certainly should know your blood type—and you have delivered and there is no obvious activity about determining whether vaccine is indicated in your case during the first few postpartum days, be sure to bring this matter up with your doctor.

Religion and Delivery

Insofar as I can determine, there is no conflict between God and childbearing or childbirth. There are, however, certain conflicting situations that arise in pregnancy and childbirth as a result of our imperfect attempts to interpret God's word. This is not meant to offend anyone. Our religious leaders agreed upon this "litany of imperfection." Our variety of faiths attests to it.

Now then, some of the very best hospitals in the world are Catholic. If I were in a strange community and sick, I would certainly go to a Catholic hospital without question. I would also go to a Baptist, Lutheran, Jewish, Presbyterian, or Methodist hospital, and so on with equal equanimity. Religious faith is not involved in my hospital decision; all the religious faiths that I am aware of run a tight ship and a good hospital.

The Catholic moral code, however, abuts rather sharply against some aspects of the management of pregnancy. In the first place, therapeutic abortion and sterilization by any means (unless the sterilization is incidental to some other procedure, say, a hysterectomy) are forbidden. But since both therapeutic abortion and sterilization are *elective* procedures, any sensible doctor would simply plan to perform them somewhere else.

The most misunderstood article in the Catholic moral code states, in part, that you can't directly take a life to save another life. For generations the following misapplication of that doctrine has been widely circulated: If, say, in the conduct of labor it becomes necessary to choose between saving a mother or her child, the child is saved and the mother allowed to die.

Now, I have practiced in a Catholic hospital for twenty-five years. During this time we have delivered close to 100,000 mothers, and not once did this supposed conflict ever arise. During the same twenty-five years, eight expectant mothers died in that hospital, most of them from nonpregnancy causes (strokes, heart disease, embolism, etc.). In no instance did anyone consider sacrificing a mother for *any* reason.

Maternal deaths must be reported. Hospital staff committees must investigate them. The worst thing an obstetrician can have on his record is a *preventable* maternal death. He must answer for his actions to his colleagues, not the Catholic hospital.

Further, hospitals are inspected at least every two years by the Joint Commission of Hospital Accreditation (JCHA). Commission members are selected from the American Hospital Association, the American Medical Association, and the American College of Surgeons. Religion has nothing to do with the JCHA. This commission inspects every aspect of hospital care; it is incredibly meticulous and thorough. Its approval is *mandatory* for a hospital to function. One of the areas inspected most closely is the maternity division. Maternal and fetal death rates, infection rates, cesarean-section rates, and many other statistics are studied. If a hospital, Catholic or not, in some way allowed a maternal death, supposedly to save an infant or for any other reason, the hospital probably would be dropped from accreditation. And so, without JCHA approval, that hospital could not have interns, residents, or nursing programs; it could not have

Medicare, Blue Cross, or any other health insurance carrier. Thus, accreditation is important—even vital—for a hospital's survival and function.

So you see that in a hospital, Catholic or not, maternal deaths are studied closely by doctors and the JCHA, and therein lies the ultimate control of our level of practice.

Another area of religious involvement has to do with blood. At one time the leading cause of maternal death was hemorrhage. For a number of reasons this is no longer true. One factor has been the constant availability of blood in modern maternity units. There are, however, some religious faiths that believe blood transfusions are forbidden by God, even the autotransfusion of a patient with her own spilled blood, a technically feasible procedure. Such limitations placed upon hospitals and doctors are so restrictive that both will often refuse to care for a patient who follows such a religion. A better solution, it appears, would be for doctor and hospital to obtain the necessary legal protection and then assume responsibility for these patients. We are all God's children.

Fascinating Facts

▷ The first cesarean section performed in the United States was carried out by John Lambert Richmond in Newton, Ohio, in 1827. Although two other doctors, Jesse Bennett of Virginia in 1794 and Francois Prevost in Donaldsville, Louisiana, in 1782, both laid claim to having performed cesarean sections, there is no adequate documentation of this. Richmond fully documented his procedure in the medical literature in 1830. The others did not and the reports are hearsay.

▷ The two most common dietary deficiencies in American mothers are iron and folic acid.

DIARY

My Seventh Month

Problems _____

Medications _____

_____

_____

Rate of baby movement on a scale of 1–10 _____

Natural childbirth classes _____

_____

_____

Special tests _____

What's going on in the world? _____

_____

_____

What's going on in my life? _____

_____

_____

My thoughts and feelings _____

_____

_____

Doctor's appointment _____

Questions To Ask

_____

_____

_____

_____

MY SEVENTH LUNAR MONTH

MY EIGHTH
LUNAR MONTH

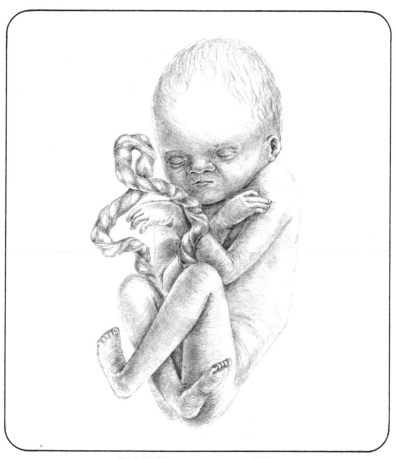

EIGHTH LUNAR MONTH

You are now entering the eighth lunar month—the twenty-eighth to thirty-second weeks. At the end of this period your baby will weigh slightly under four pounds (1800 grams), and from the crown of its head to the tip of its rump (C–R distance) it measures about 11.2 inches (28 cm), and will be kicking actively—as indeed it is now—in your throat, your side, and over your bladder, all at the same time, it seems. The reason you can feel movement in so many places simultaneously is that your baby is suspended, weightless, completely surrounded by water, like a skin diver, and it can move all four extremities at the same time. Also, your baby often has spontaneous rhythmic contractions of its diaphragm, which, for want of a better description, resemble hiccups. When you are lying still you can feel these regular jerking movements. Your baby's skin is parchment thin and the blood vessels can be seen coursing through it in a very, very fine fanlike pattern. Your baby can see and hear, but there aren't really very many chances to use these finely tuned capabilities. However, your baby now recognizes your voice.

Premature Rupture of the Membrane (PROM)

This not uncommon obstetrical complication occurs when the amniotic membranes break prior to the onset of labor, that is, prior to progressive dilation and thinning of the cervix. At or approaching full term PROM does not create a very serious problem, since about 95 percent of the time, spontaneous labor follows shortly thereafter. If it does not, induction or in some situations cesarean section may be resorted to. Whatever the method used to effect labor and delivery, a mature child is what results, and we move on to the next problem—raising it!

On the other hand, PROM is a very serious problem when it involves a preterm pregnancy. It puts both the expectant mother and her infant in significant jeopardy and is many times a very difficult and dangerous obstetrical problem to manage.

While PROM occurs in 10 percent of all pregnancies, only one in five of these are truly premature pregnancies as determined by fetal size and by dates. Regardless of what is done in these cases, 70 percent deliver within three days. Sometimes that is good, sometimes bad. Sometimes the baby is better off in the uterus, sometimes it is better off in an incubator. It depends.

This fairly common complication is caused by several situations, most commonly by increased intrauterine pressure with resistance of the uterus to further expansion and by certain types of bacterial infections found at the back of the vagina. When PROM occurs, labor, abnormal presentation of the infant, infection (amnionitis), cord prolapse, or respiratory distress syndrome in the infant (RDS) may follow.

Assessing the current fetal status is the first step in managing premature rupture of the membrane. Evidence of the degree of fetal maturity is sought by rechecking the clinical dates, doing repeated ultrasound examinations, and taking a transabdominal amniocentesis sample to determine fetal lung maturity. Further assessment of the fetus would include observation and studies for potential infection. Such things as maternal fever, increased fetal heart rate, and amniotic fluid abnormalities would tend to indicate incipient infection.

Once the fetal status is determined, the decision must be made of whether to effect delivery at once. If delivery is not indicated, there are numerous ways of attempting to prevent premature labor, as you will see in the next section. Sometimes these are very successful.

However, with premature rupture of the membrane in the presence of infection or certain other complications, it is not wise to halt labor. In fact, the reverse may be true. That is, it may be better to have the child delivered and in a safer environment—an incubator. Sometimes cortisone and other steroid agents are given during the latent period before labor begins, to try to increase the maturity of the infant's lungs, and sometimes antibiotics are given to try to arrest infection. Resolving whether or not to use these agents requires a great deal of skill and judgment, and each particular case must be treated individually. As always, what has been said here is a broad general outline of the problem and the various modes of treatment that may or may not be entered into. Again, your own doctor will know the best way to proceed in this matter if it should happen to befall you.

Prematurity and Premature Labor

About one of every ten to twelve pregnancies ends prematurely. This, therefore, is a vastly important area of obstetrics, since it can cause a great deal of fetal loss, damaged survivors, and personal heartbreak. Believe it or not, premature birth is one of the leading causes of all deaths in the United States. Add to this the problem of disadvantaged infants and their cost to society and to you, and you begin to become aware of the magnitude of the problem.

First of all, what is considered a premature birth? Well, in terms of size, an infant whose weight at birth is 2500 grams (5 lbs., 8 oz. or less) is deemed premature. In terms of time, any child born before the thirty-seventh week is considered premature. Neither statistical guideline is entirely satisfactory, and thus any child born early or small and as a result unable to cope with life outside the uterus may be called premature. We have seen this fact in our discussion of intrauterine growth retardation in chapter 6. We also note that in some societies ethnic differences result in smaller babies because of the genetic constitution of that society. Therefore, it is difficult to make any comparisons of survival or treatment that stand up in different ethnic groups and countries.

What causes prematurity and premature labor? Well, there are a great number of causes. Many of them are interrelated and many are not. In the first place, we as doctors create a certain amount of prematurity when we induce labor in certain medical conditions already noted elsewhere in the book. Thus, hypertension of pregnancy, IUGR, diabetes, Rh disorders, and so on may lead us to empty the uterus early since the fetus is no longer safe within it. We have also contributed to prematurity by doing repeat elective cesarean sections prior to full maturity. These procedures do occur in the best regulated practices but are now a very minor contribution to prematurity.

Having put those factors aside, let us look at the most common causes of prematurity.

- malnutrition
- very young and very old mothers
- premature rupture of the membranes
- tobacco, alcohol, and drugs
- maternal disease—diabetes, hypertension, renal disorders, etc
- abnormal uterine size or shape, such as found in the presence of tumors or congenital malformations
- multiple pregnancy
- weakness of the cervix (incompetent cervical os)
- abnormal placental location or premature separation of the placenta

What are the problems that prematurity brings to the little ones? Well, it's like a blast-off before the astronaut has put on his space suit, buckled down, or attached his oxygen line. Our newborn's lungs aren't ready to breathe (really the worst problem); its temperature-control mechanism is weak; its digestive, excretory, and enzyme systems are all not quite "go." It doesn't have sufficient fat deposits to help insulate against temperature changes. But blast-off has occurred, so what do we do?

First, labor must be managed most carefully; pain-relief measures should be those least likely to depress the baby. Monitoring of fetal activity and well-being should be continued throughout labor and delivery. Following delivery, immediate transfer to an intensive-care nursery follows. This is the best environment to minimize the effects of respiratory distress syndrome (RDS), the most likely opponent of the baby's well-being, and to minimize the other critical problems that may befall it. Dramatic improvement in the survival rate of small prematures is now the order of the day, as is the quality of their survival. All this is due to modern intensive-care nurseries and neonatologists or very highly skilled pediatricians.

Prevention of premature labor is the best solution for all these problems. However, this is very difficult to achieve, since success mainly rests with prenatal care and compliance. Sometimes there is nothing that can be done to help a malnourished mother-to-be, although in our society today, with all the assistance that is provided, it would seem that much malnourishment of an expectant mother must be self-induced, whether the expectant mother is rich or poor.

Some of the other deviations from sense—the use of tobacco, alcohol, and drugs—are also self-induced. Proper sex education and protection to avoid pregnancy in the very young would reduce prematurity very significantly. Further, the control of maternal diseases such as diabetes, high blood pressure, and so forth, and the close monitoring of older expectant mothers—all will help. Avoiding premature rupture of the membrane is difficult, but our greater understanding of vaginal infections and their relationship to premature rupture of the membrane helps in this area. And so we see that in all these areas, control of the conditions that cause premature labor represents our key to success.

Once premature labor has become established, there are three general medical programs that are used with varying success to arrest labor.

- Ritodrine is now FDA approved for use in the control of premature labor. It is a very powerful and dangerous drug that must be used only in institutions quite capable of handling it and certain potential complications to the mother, particularly her cardiovascular system. Generally it is administered intravenously at the beginning of premature labor and, if successful, the oral route is used for long-term treatment.
- Magnesium sulfate has been and is indeed still used for the control of hypertension of pregnancy. But one of its further properties is that of a uterine muscle relaxant, and so it is also used to prevent premature labor, particularly in those patients in which it is unsafe to use Ritodrine. Magnesium sulfate is also administered intravenously in the beginning, and then the mode of administration may be switched at a later time.
- Alcohol—intravenously, not orally—has been used to control acute premature labor. It obviously cannot be used for long periods of time, and it is generally being discarded in most institutions at this time as an agent for arresting premature labor.

Again, all these drugs are exceedingly active and have profound effects upon the expectant mother and the fetus. They must be and they are used judiciously according to strict protocols, and the benefits and risks must be weighed by you and your doctor together before institution.

Perinatology

Some mention has been made previously of perinatologists, but a little more elaboration at this time won't hurt. The specialty is also called perinatal medicine and, more lately, maternal-fetal medicine. There are very few such doctors in the world today, but their numbers are growing rapidly and they now comprise a recognized subspecialty of obstetrics.

The tools of perinatology include some of the fetologist's equipment—amniocentesis, for instance. The perinatologist further studies maternal health, nutrition, and body functions, particularly in high-risk mothers. Using electronic and laboratory monitoring, he or she observes growth and development of the baby, gauges placental reserve, and, finally, intensively monitors both mother and child during labor and delivery, with all the equipment and judgment available.

Neonatology

This subspecialty also needs a little more elaboration at this period, although it really belongs to the field of pediatrics. The neonatologist is highly specialized to take care of endangered newborns in an intensive-care nursery—which, incidentally, resembles the flight deck of a spaceship. There are instruments to measure everything; to eat for, breathe for, heat—everything except fondle—sick newborns till they can make it on their own. Thus very premature babies, or those from high-risk mothers, or the products of difficult labors or deliveries—distressed babies from whatever cause—can enter this intensive-care environment and be ministered to with the specialized skills of a neonatologist and stand an excellent chance of survival undamaged.

Metabolic Changes in Late Pregnancy

During these last few months your basal metabolic rate (the rate at which fuel—sugar—is burned by oxygen in your body) increases. This rise persists until your delivery, at which time it drops very rapidly to slightly below normal and stays there for several months. These changes in metabolism cause you to have more energy during late pregnancy, but they also decrease your tolerance of heat and your ability to sleep. If your last trimester happens to fall in the summertime, it can be very uncomfortable indeed. Insomnia, for this and many other reasons, is even more common now, and sleep becomes a precious commodity. Turn up the air conditioner and get a two-foot-wide blanket for your husband.

Pain Again

Numerous little localities in your anatomy now begin to ache, puff, crack, turn up, turn down, turn out, bend, swell, hurt, sag, explode, get numb, and get sore.

Rib Pain

Your growing little one is pushing everything that used to be in your lower abdomen into your upper abdomen and everything that was in your upper abdomen into your chest. As a result, your rib cage has to expand, the lower ribs frequently separating spontaneously from the breastbone (sternum). These free-floating ribs can produce considerable local discomfort, particularly on your right side. The discomfort continues off and on until you have delivered, at which time the rib cage closes again and the separated members rejoin the breastbone. Like so many of the burdens you have to bear at this time, nothing can be done to prevent or correct rib separation. Everything has got to be somewhere.

Pressure Pain

At the other end of the line, your precious passenger packs the bladder, the rectum, and all the pelvic organs into a waferlike compress of agonized organs. This produces a significant amount of lower abdominal discomfort, bladder and rectal pressure, pressure transmitted into the back, down the legs, and so on. Sometimes wearing a supportive maternity girdle, which raises the infant out of your lower abdomen helps. Generally, it just pushes the load farther under your ribs, with predictable results up above.

Braxton Hicks Contractions

During the third month of pregnancy, your uterus begins to contract rhythmically in order to help circulate blood. The contractions continue throughout pregnancy and are usually painless. You may describe to your doctor that the baby is knotting up in your abdomen, though of course it is not the baby but the muscles of the uterus that produce the sensation. (This same knotting occurs during labor, but then, because of certain differences in what is going on, pain is produced.) Occasionally these early contractions, named after the obstetrician who first described them, are painful, and occasionally they produce false labor. There is no danger that Braxton Hicks contractions, even though painful, will produce real labor. When they annoy you too much, mix yourself a relaxing drink and lie down. Read in chapter 10 how you can identify false labor and differentiate it from the real thing.

Numb Spots

Although numbness cannot generally be equated with pain, it is still an unpleasant sensation, and pregnancy produces its own little points of numbness. One popular area is the abdomen, which, as it expands, stretches superficial nerve fibers that spread out to cover the skin. As a result, certain areas in the upper abdomen and over the lower rib cage often become numb and occasionally become exquisitely sensitive.

Likewise, it is not uncommon to have numbness and tingling in your fingers in the last few months of pregnancy. This is produced by swelling of the supportive tissue tunnels that carry the major nerve trunks into the arms and hands. The condition is called the carpal tunnel syndrome. Diuretics (water pills) can perhaps reduce the swelling in such tissue tunnels, but they are not very successful and certainly are not to be recommended during pregnancy.

Although no permanent damage has been clearly demonstrated by this carpal tunnel syndrome during pregnancy, it has occurred in certain other medical situations in which some nerve disability has followed, and so it would be well for you to at least advise your doctor of this sensation.

Umbilical Hernia

There generally exists a little defect in the abdominal cavity around the area of your navel (umbilicus) that is significant to you only during pregnancy. This defective spot can sometimes fill with tissue from inside the abdominal cavity and become quite tender. The hernias thus formed can be reduced or pushed back, and your doctor will show you how. The problem disappears as soon as delivery takes place.

Nursing

Colostrum (the forerunner of milk) may now seep regularly from the nipples, and it can stain just about everything. The breast changes that were detailed earlier mostly continue. The area around the nipple, the areola, generally becomes even darker, and striae keep cracking away at your outer skin.

197

Nursing a baby is not a recordable event, so statistics are hard to come by concerning the frequency of its occurrence. However, in the 1960s apparently this normal, wonderful physiological event was happening after about 18 to 20 percent of all pregnancies. Since then the percentage of mothers who are breast-feeding has increased rapidly, and probably half of all new mothers are at least interested and are trying to nurse. And in some areas of the country, such as southern California, the percentage is well over 75 percent. If you are planning on nursing—and you should if you can, and most of you will be able to—it is important that when you massage your breasts with lanolin skin cream, you make sure the nipples are soft and supple. If your nipples tend to be inverted or withdrawn, you should strip them outward and pull on them so that they will stand out well when baby begins to nurse. But you don't have to move to southern California!

Shortly after delivery, it is quite common for the breasts to become very engorged, tender, and uncomfortable. This, you may have been told, is when the milk comes in. Although that statement may be true, the engorgement is not due to milk itself but to congestion and fluid (edema) accumulating in the breast tissue. At one time hormone substances were given to control this, but most often that is not the case nowadays. Do not worry about your ability to make milk, because if you do, there probably will be no milk—a self-fulfilling prophecy.

Although the substitute formulas now available seem to be generally very adequate, there is still nothing that approaches the quality of natural mother's milk. The decision of whether to nurse involves many variables. You may feel that if you are going back to work as soon as possible after you deliver, there is no point in trying to nurse. This is probably not so. On the other hand, if you are planning on nursing because of pressure placed on you by family or friends or fads, or what you have read, there is no point in nursing at all. You have already lost your greatest psychological advantage. If you have had a complicated pregnancy or labor or delivery, which has drained you of your resources, it would be damaging to you and probably to the baby for you to nurse. This is also true, of course, if you have certain systemic illnesses.

To nurse is to complete the natural human cycle of pregnancy, delivery, and child-rearing. If it is your wish and if you are able, nursing is of great psychological benefit to both you and your child, and you should do it. On the other hand, as we have already noted, if it is not your wish to nurse and you do so because of outside pressure or because you feel you should, the nursing procedure will become a burden surrounded by tension, apprehension, and disenchantment. Your baby will very rapidly sense this, and the result will be more harmful than good for your relationship. You yourself should make the decision of whether to nurse after reviewing the available information and assessing your own wishes, values, and desires.

Here follows a list of some information and some more or less known facts about the pros and cons of breast-feeding:

• Breast-feeding is not advisable when the mother is a hepatitis B carrier, if she is severely ill with a systemic disorder, or if she is markedly anemic. It may also not be recommended if she has active toxoplasmosis or cytomegalovirus, or is on hard drugs or dangerous medication or smokes excessively.
• Recent studies reveal that the presence of lymphocytes, antibodies, and other proteins in the mother's milk can protect babies from a great number of communicable and infectious complications. Thus breast-fed babies may be protected from killers like sudden infant death syndrome (SIDS) and necrotizing enterocolitis.
• More bottle-fed infants die in epidemics of gastroenteritis than do breast-fed babies.
• Human milk contains a substance, lactoferrin, that inhibits the growth of certain pathological bacteria in the intestines.
• Breast-fed babies have less allergy and less ear disease, and

never have calcium-deficiency muscle spasms.

• Cow's milk contains more sodium and chloride than does human milk. This may produce dehydration, particularly if solid foods are introduced too early.

• Mother's milk contains a substance that triggers baby's appetite-control mechanism. The breast-fed baby then is less likely to be an obese baby. Obese babies become obese adults.

• Animal milk may become contaminated if sterile precautions are not observed. Human milk may be contaminated, as noted in the first item of this list.

• Breast-feeding, if enjoyed, is psychologically better for both participants.

• And it is cheaper.

• Hormones are very seldom used after delivery to suppress lactation. Certain medications are given to mothers who cannot or will not nurse, but generally they are not hormone substances, and they must usually be taken for a fairly long period of time.

If you wish to know more about breast-feeding, check the phone book for the La Lêche League in your community.

Milk

Mention has been made before about the good and bad in cow's milk, but let's get it all together here.

• Normally infants produce enough lactase until age two to handle all the milk they can get. Thereafter, lactase levels drop rapidly. Lactase is the enzyme that digests milk sugar—lactose. It is safe to say, then, that milk, particularly human milk, is good baby food. After two years of age, people and milk should probably begin to part company. Here's why:

About 50 million Americans (1 in 4) cannot tolerate lactose (milk sugar) because of low lactase levels in their bodies.

Milk gives these adults and older children cramps, bloating, fullness, and occasionally diarrhea.

Further, if milk, in any quantity, is consumed, lactose intolerance can interfere with carbohydrate and, possibly, protein metabolism.

True milk allergy occurs in up to 7 percent of the population, and its ingestion produces allergic reactions of various kinds and severity.

- Yogurt—milk that has been naturally fermented with lactobacillus—has had most of its lactose inactivated or hydrolyzed. It is, therefore, safe food for lactose-intolerant and milk-allergic people. However, most commercial yogurt is not so prepared. Read the label.
- Adults should restrict milk intake (even if they can drink it) to one pint of skim milk a day. This is because milk, particularly whole milk and more particularly homogenized milk, is rich in cholesterol, a prime mover in heart disease.
- Pregnant women (and newborn babies) who drink cow's milk can have calcium-deficiency muscle spasms. This is because calcium absorption from cow's milk is blocked by other substances present in such milk. We have already seen that newborns on mother's milk do not have this problem. Expectant mothers get their muscle symptoms in the form of early-morning leg cramps.
- Standard pregnancy diets have traditionally included at least one quart of milk daily (but your diet does not). Studies show that lactose-intolerant pregnant women (1 in 4, remember) who are forced to consume at least one quart of milk daily have significantly smaller babies than pregnant women who do not drink milk.

The Placenta

This piece of equipment, commonly called the afterbirth, is made by your baby and belongs to your baby. It connects you to each other by partially invading the inner surface of your uterus. Why you don't reject it (since it is a transplant from another human being) and why it stops invading your body at the point which it does have been the subject of much study and considerable theorizing. Very rarely, the placenta can go wild and invade its host (you) and cause what was once the most fatal of all cancers; fortunately it is now curable.

At full term a placenta is a bloody, spongy, pie-shape organ weighing about two pounds, with membranes trailing off its edges. Here are some other interesting details:

- It has a life span of about nine months. It dies, of course, at birth, and under the microscope it shows all the signs of old age—including hardening of the arteries!
- There is tremendous "reserve" in normal placentas. This reserve is to protect the baby in cases of partial detachment of the placenta or in cases in which placental senescence or premature aging robs the fetus of necessary food and oxygen and thus produces distress.
- Your baby's blood is pumped back and forth through the umbilical cord and filtered by the placenta. It never normally comes directly in touch with your blood but, as in a heart-lung machine, is always separated by a membrane of sorts. It is true, as you have seen in the Rh disorders, that small spurts of fetal blood can escape into the maternal circulation, particularly in late pregnancy, but these are very minor connections indeed. Bathing on one side of this membrane, baby pulls food and oxygen over from you through the blood—plus alcohol, nicotine, medicine, drugs—whatever happens to be floating past at the time. In return, baby slips you carbon dioxide and other waste products for you to

eliminate. So you are eating for two and excreting for two—though of course one is very small.

- The placenta secretes a number of hormones that trigger all sorts of responses, both locally and around your body. Mainly it produces chorionic gonadotropin (which makes pregnancy tests positive, breasts grow, menstruation stop, and so on), progesterone (which allows the uterus to grow and not expel the baby until the time comes), and certain other hormones and enzymes, some of which can have powerful systemic effects on your blood pressure, metabolism, breasts, lactation, etc.

- New discoveries of substances called prostaglandins throughout our bodies have yielded information about the onset of labor. The placenta, it appears, is programmed to secrete a certain prostaglandin in large amounts during its dying days. This prostaglandin can overcome all uterine relaxants and protectants and so labor begins. But it is not really quite that simple. Other things are involved in the onset of labor.

- Most placentas are discarded at birth, but occasionally one ends up in the laboratory if it appears unusual in any important way or is needed as part of a specific research program. Moreover, some pharmaceutical companies in the United States buy placentas and use them in order to extract certain very specific and powerful hormones, which they use either in research or in hormone manufacturing. They don't pay very much for the used placentas, so don't expect a cut in your hospital bill.

Newborn Insurance

Practically all fifty states now have legislation that requires all family health-insurance policies to cover newborns from the moment of birth. Until recently most family insurance policies were written to cover the costs for treatment of newborn illness or defects, but some did not cover the first fourteen to thirty days.

The new laws cover any baby for any illness or complication needing treatment from the moment he or she is born.

Contact your insurance agent and make sure your policy covers newborns (but to make this part of your policy effective you must notify your insurance carrier within thirty days of your baby's birth, providing baby's birth date, name, sex, and parents' insurance policy number).

Preparation for Childbirth

First, about pain. I have just finished reading a fascinating newspaper column by a very well known and highly respected writer. Her theme was that women for the most part are dumb and stupid because millions of them conceived each year against their wishes, simply because they failed to use simple, readily available birth control methods. She herself is a liberated American woman who speaks freely and regularly on these matters. She is highly regarded by other women. I wonder, however, what would happen to me had *I* written the same column. Probably the same fate that would befall someone making a third-party entrance into a husband-wife quarrel!

And so it is that a man has some meaningful hesitation—if he has any sense—before making any remarks concerning pain in childbearing. I have participated (as much as possible) in many thousands of deliveries, both before and after preparedness, before and after deep sleep (also called twilight), and before and after epidurals; delivering babies in hospitals, homes, taxis, airplanes, trains, bathrooms—you name it. I thus at least have a feeling for the subject I am about to address.

No one can gain access to the past or to anything that precedes our own moment of time except through history. Historical records, unfortunately, yield just about any version of what we seek on any given subject. For example, if you read

204

the American version of our revolution and then read the British version, you come away believing that they were describing two separate and distinct conflicts. Having thus prepared my way by cutting up the boards and nailing my coffin together, I will proceed to tell you my thoughts and views on the pain and peril of childbearing, and what history has taught me.

It is best that we not use the term *natural childbirth*, as was coined by Dr. Grantly Dick Read in the original work on preparation for childbearing. Natural childbirth to me denotes what took place prior to the scientific era of obstetrics. During those times many women conceived and delivered without difficulty. Because of natural selection, the weak and the deformed died without being able to finish the reproductive act. Further, those with any severe obstetrical problem or complication, no matter how strong they may have been, died with their babies. This was, and still is, the law of nature in any other species but the human, and that is truly "natural childbirth" and nature's way.

It is very true that when physicians began assisting in the birthing chamber, they committed many errors, and many women and their children suffered while doctors were learning the specialty so long denied them. However, as a result of these pioneer efforts, a high level of safety for mother and child has finally been achieved, to the point that some people, with a false sense of security generated by hospital safety, have chosen to separate themselves and deliver away from this unnatural environment that we have created. But more on this later. I digress, and we need to get back to pain.

- There is no "curse of Eve." Women were not and are not destined or ordained to bring forth in pain and sorrow.
- Even disregarding very abnormal obstructed labor, there is no assurance that pain is not attendant upon a normal delivery. Pain-producing events occur during normal labor, and I have seen them a multitude of times, time after time.

If, however, pain sensation is not perceived by the laboring mother, then a block of pain stimulation must arise from within by unknown mechanisms—mechanisms that have always been present and are unrelated to any enlightenment or preparation.

- Doctors did not introduce pain in childbearing. One does not have to rely on history or historians to confirm that fact. There are plenty of areas in our world today where that fact can be confirmed—if you have a strong stomach and wish to make the trip. The doctor's role has not been to make pain and fear but to treat them—and so they did, starting in a society that was not mature enough to accept anything but some kind of sedation. It was, after all, doctors—male doctors—who, released from the constant combat with death and disability in the early delivery chambers, first developed the concept of mature preparedness for childbirth, thus releasing patients from sedation. Regular obstetricians may have been slow in accepting the new concepts but *so were their patients.* Thus doctors who moved forward too fast left their patients behind and so had no practice at all. I was one of them! An average physician attempting to introduce a new concept, however good, may lose his practice and more. And if a doctor accepts, without deliberation, every new thought that someone else perceives to be of value, we would all be in constant trouble. (Like birthing babies underwater, for instance!)

- The introduction of techniques for the prepared childbirth experience marked a giant step forward in obstetrical care. Not only did it reduce or obliterate the need for depressant medications during labor, it enhanced the whole birth experience for everyone involved—mother, father, siblings, and attendants.

The modern era of prepared childbirth began in the 1950s with the publication of Grantly Dick Read's work (*Childbirth*

Without Fear) on natural childbirth. The essence of his philosophy was that bearing and delivering a child is a normal physiological experience, and that with proper preparation, knowledge, and the absence of fear, pain should be minimal. And it became so, at least for most of the women in the program.

However, the Read fervor gradually dissipated, although classes for expectant parents continued, and training exercises continued. In time various other programs became more popular. Today the Lamaze program and its variations are undoubtedly the most popular approaches to planned labor and delivery. Fundamentally, Dr. Lamaze felt that women should be prepared emotionally and psychologically for childbearing, in accordance with Pavlov's principle of the conditioned response. This principle, which has been called psychoprophylaxis, states that the brain can be trained to accept a given stimulus and select its response. As applied to childbearing, Lamaze believed that women could be trained to respond in a *positive* fashion to the contractions of their uterus during labor and delivery, and also to the attendant stretching of the tissues throughout the birth canal and vagina at the time of delivery.

There are as many varieties of the Lamaze approach to conditioning for labor as there are teachers, and the American method differs from the French and Russian versions. The basic philosophy, however, remains unchanged. It is not necessarily childbirth without pain, nor is it necessarily childbirth without anesthesia; it is positive conditioning used as training for the birth experience.

Here are some points to ponder:

- Education for childbirth is a magnificent concept *when it remains factual.* Knowledge diminishes fear and increases cooperation. The need for—indeed the desire for—drugs is diminished. It becomes a joyful experience, and I heartily recommend it to you.
- Educated childbirth is not *natural* childbirth, however, since

it requires learning procedures and techniques that not only alter the environment but that are sometimes impossible for some women to master.

- The need for anesthetic support in any type of prepared delivery should not be regarded as a failure of the technique or of the mother; nor should it be attended by any sense of shame or guilt by the bearing mother, or fear for her child's safety or health. One of the sad disadvantages of any of these techniques is that it may be in the hands of an overzealous teacher who believes and teaches that everyone should win the gold. This in turn produces a sense of failure and shame among the other medalists. All you need to do is your very best.

- When both prospective participants are in agreement, it is altogether desirable for a husband, live-in mate, or close friend to participate in the labor and delivery process and, indeed, in the classes. Only then should it be done. Some partners get see-sick and frightened. Moreover, there are some men who find that the degree of intimacy involved in sharing this fundamental experience is more than they can reasonably and positively deal with. Consequently, for them the affair is neither fulfilling nor rewarding; nor does it increase their ability to be intimate in any future relationship. Indeed, for some the reverse is true, and with this participation, particularly when it is forced upon them by peer or other pressures, they may become more detached, with long-term negative psychological consequences for the relationship. The last word has not been written on these and the other social and interpersonal changes in our time, nor has their long-term effect—good or bad—been determined or their influence on marriage, divorce, the family setting, and unity as well as upon child development. Indeed, present social statistics are sufficiently wretched and melancholy to make us wonder if we are doing anything right.

Altered Hospital Settings

Let's get back to this subject. The strict hospital rules that once isolated laboring women from their families and friends were instituted by physicians generations ago, in order to reduce the risk of infection and for a number of other reasons that no longer exist. To pry us out of this long-casted mold required a good deal of consumer pressure, and this turned out to be an altogether good and rewarding reaction. Women had been denied the company of their loved ones during labor or denied preparation for childbirth and a warm laboring environment. Women eventually revolted and started moving back toward home deliveries. This movement has gained momentum over the past decade, and while it is an altogether pleasant way to have a normal delivery, it is a treacherous environment, as our past reveals and documents so clearly. Not wishing to delve into that controversial subject any deeper now (see Home Births, chapter 9), since my views must be clear to all, I want to discuss briefly the effects this movement has had upon the hospital environment.

In most hospitals now offering obstetrical care, birthing rooms and modified delivery rooms are appearing. In a typical birthing room the furnishings are those of an average bedroom, with most of the obstetrical equipment blocked from view by a variety of mechanisms. In such a setting women may labor in a homelike environment, with their family and friends present as their wishes dictate, with a bed that can be broken apart during the time of delivery so that the doctor has easy access to carry out the delivery procedures. In the event that some unforeseen complication develops, all the facilities the hospital can marshal are readily available, either in a sectioned-off area of the bedroom or in a nearby delivery suite. All the hospital laboratory facilities and anesthesia capabilities are also close by.

Hospitals are now sponsoring not only prepared childbirth

classes but parenting, sibling, and nursing classes that involve the family as a unit, and they have almost always met with great acceptance by the community *and* the medical profession. Many times it is possible to labor and deliver in one of these birthing centers and be sent on home a few hours after delivery without ever having been admitted to the hospital. But there are great advantages to just being there.

Fascinating Facts

▷ A recent study by a group of psychologists shows that the risk of premature delivery was doubled for both white and black women when a positive pregnancy anticipation was combined with high or rising levels of distress. Conversely, both groups experienced a slight decrease in premature labor despite an anxiety-producing life-style if there also existed a low pregnancy desirability! Figure that out!

▷ The fetus within you can hear what goes on outside, so you may want to watch your language. There is ample evidence that it already knows your voice and recognizes it at the time of birth. That's why it may turn to you when placed on your abdomen following delivery. It is also becoming clear that behavioral patterns and traits characteristic of each child exist in the uterus from about the twenty-eighth week on and may be well enough established to predict some characteristics of the newborn.

DIARY

My Eighth Month

Problems _____

Medications _____

_____

_____

Illness _____

_____

_____

Rate of baby movement on a scale of 1–10 _____

Special tests _____

Natural childbirth classes _____

_____

_____

What's going on in the world? _____

_____

_____

_____

What's going on in my life? _____

_____

_____

_____

My thoughts and feelings _____

_____

_____

Doctor's appointment _____

Questions To Ask

_____

_____

_____

_____

_____

_____

_____

_____

_____

_____

_____

_____

_____

_____

_____

_____

_____

_____

_____

_____

_____

_____

_____

_____

CHAPTER NINE

MY NINTH
LUNAR MONTH

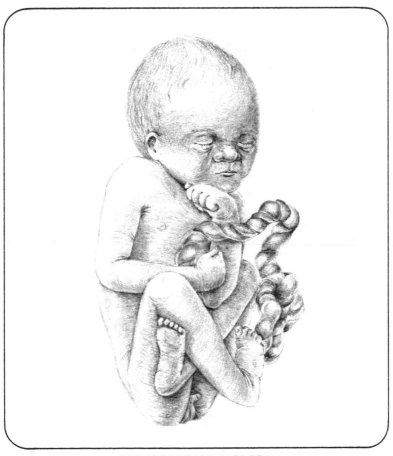

NINTH LUNAR MONTH

You are now in the ninth month of your pregnancy—but
you know that better than anyone else. This comprises
the thirty-second to the thirty-sixth weeks. At the end of this
period your baby weighs between five and six pounds (2400–
2700 grams) and is about eighteen inches long (47 cms), but
the C–R measurement is 13.6 inches (34 cms). The C–R length,
mentioned on page 188, is often used in place of total body
length. There now is a good deal of fat deposited under the
skin to protect the vital organs from temperature changes. A
baby born at this time will survive as well as one delivered at
term and will be going home with you unless some unexpected
complication occurs.

Speaking of home, you probably have made everything ready
for your guest, packed and repacked your bag, and had several
dry runs to the hospital. You have had ten baby showers and
received thirty baby outfits all of which will fit the first week
after birth only. All you need now is a little more patience.

Home Births

In recent years there has been an increased interest in home
deliveries, although this interest has apparently not increased
the rate of occurrence of such events, as you will see. Multiple
factors, some of which you know about already, have been
responsible for this renewed interest in an old custom. For
instance:

- Rage and anger against a restrictive hospital system that was too slow in responding to the perceived needs of a more liberal and enlightened society. Having all but conquered maternal mortality and having made vast inroads on fetal loss, doctors and hospitals were slow in surrendering absolute control over the environment and policies that had achieved this remarkable goal. At the same time, similar anger was expressed by the new generation against most organized societal institutions. This anger reached maximum expression in the sixties and seventies, when many dissident citizens did indeed drop out and form their own colonies. Not many of these exist anymore, and certainly, insofar as our own institutions are concerned, the hospital environment has vastly changed and is very responsive to the family unit.

- Costs. Having a baby delivered within the system today is an expensive event, no question about it. Here are the American averages: for the hospital—$2,209.10; for the doctor—$623.50; for the anesthesia—$150; for the pediatrician—$64.00. Again, these are averages for a normal delivery and include only a two-day hospital stay. Against these figures is the cost of a midwife at home—$715.70. Some of our citizens—and aliens—have no money at all and certainly not enough for either system—not for a delivery at the hospital or for a midwife at home. Statistics reveal that depressed areas of our country with a high alien population have the highest number of home deliveries.

- Back-to-nature faddism. It is now "in" to have a baby at home, and some of your best friends are doing it and the subject usually comes up for discussion at parties just after football and basketball but before car pooling and divorces.

- Speed. Some very rapid fire mothers just don't make it in time and, of course, in certain remote or weather-bound areas of our country the time it takes to get to a hospital is too great.

Here are some further facts and figures about home births.

- The number of out-of-hospital births in the United States has remained more or less constant since 1975. This figure is about 1 percent, and it varies considerably across the United States. In Connecticut and North Dakota $\frac{2}{10}$ of a percent of all deliveries are home births, as compared to Texas with 3 percent, Washington state with 3.5 percent, and Oregon with 4.4 percent. The reasons for these variables seem clear.
- Home births are *not* underreported. If anything they are overreported so that noncitizens can get U.S. citizenship for their children.
- About one-third of home deliveries are attended by midwives, about a third by physicians, and a third by unspecified persons.
- As the percentage of hospital births has risen, so have infant deaths and maternal deaths declined. In 1940, for instance, when 56 percent of all deliveries occurred in hospitals, the infant mortality rate was 47 per thousand and the maternal death rate 376 per hundred thousand. In 1980, 99 percent of all deliveries were in hospitals, the infant mortality rate was 12.4 per thousand, and the maternal mortality rate 6.9 per hundred thousand!
- Figures from the National Center on Health Statistics show that 20 percent of women with *no underlying medical conditions* and no previous problem with pregnancy develop some problem during labor.
- It is a myth to say that other developed countries have most of their births out of the hospital. In Great Britain, for instance, 98.5 percent of all births occur in hospitals. In Holland, another country often quoted as having low infant and maternal mortality rates and a high home birth rate, the percentage of hospital deliveries is now over 60 percent and is steadily increasing. The women who stay home in Holland are low-risk women who have no other choice, since the

216

government will not pay for their use of hospital facilities.

- The belief that childbirth is so safe it can take place anywhere, or the opposite, that all births outside the hospital are unsafe, are probably both untrue. But of the 20 percent of laboring women who in a previously normal pregnancy undergo pathological events while they are laboring or delivering, 2 percent represent *acute* problems requiring *immediate* solutions. As an example, shoulder disproportion is not an uncommon delivery event. The head delivers but the shoulders are trapped and require expert management to deliver with safety to both mother and child, a situation that allows little time leeway. A further example would be a prolapsed cord, which is also not an uncommon event that will destroy the child within minutes if aggressive treatment is not instituted.

My feelings have probably shown through in this presentation. If you can afford it or are insured, I believe you should go to a family-oriented hospital or birthing center to have your baby. If you cannot, you should have a good midwife or physician and be in reasonably close proximity to a well-run maternity hospital.

Gravida ... Para ...

You will hear of or read about doctors categorizing pregnant women as *gravida* something *para* something. It sounds very confusing, but it's very simple. *Gravid* or *gravida* refers to the total number of pregnancies one woman has sustained, whether they were full term, premature, abortions, or ectopics. No matter; each pregnancy raises gravida by one. *Para—parity* or *parous—* refers to the number of viable deliveries the gravida has sustained. Thus a woman who is "gravida four para two" (G_4P_2) has been pregnant four times, with two viable deliveries. This is of little use to you, perhaps, but it has some value to us doctors. We use the abbreviators in writing case reports, communicating with other physicians, and in keeping hospital records.

Late Examinations by Your Doctor

During the last weeks of your pregnancy, your doctor may examine you internally and may do so more than once. At this time the size of your pelvis is reevaluated so as to further determine whether its capacity is sufficient to allow passage of your baby's head. One of the reasons this is repeated in late pregnancy is that the baby's head, which is normally the largest part to go through your pelvis, is usually now presenting within the pelvis or close to it. The examination assists in many ways to help evaluate whether your internal measurements are adequate to accept it. Also at this time the opportunity is present to determine whether the head is in normal position and is coming down well and deep into your pelvis. Finally, such an examination provides an opportunity to evaluate how close to labor you may be. Often the doctor can tell by the condition of your cervix whether labor is imminent or a long way off. Generally, prior to the onset of labor the cervix begins to thin and to open and soften. Sometimes, however, labor begins when the cervix is most unfavorable and unripe.

These late examinations are quite a common and accepted procedure in modern obstetrics. Occasionally you may spot for many hours afterward, but this should cause no alarm. Very rarely you may actually bleed, and if this persists or is increasing over a period of several hours, you had better check back.

Admission to the Hospital

Hospitals shouldn't frighten you, particularly modern obstetrical units, and certainly those that are family centered and allow free visitation during and after labor. As you already know, the day of closed, off-limits delivery suites and of sadistic obstetrical attendants has long since passed. Perhaps you have already toured your own obstetrical unit with your prepared childbirth classes and you are aware that what I am saying is true. If you have not done so, you should.

What to Bring

- a suitcase containing your nightgowns, robe, slippers
- your personal toilet articles—comb, brush, toothbrush, makeup
- cigarettes and matches, if you still smoke—but if you are sharing a room be considerate of your roommate
- nursing bras and bed jacket
- writing paper, thank-you notepaper, and a pen
- an outfit for your baby to wear home (a diaper is not necessary)
- the baby's father!

If baby is on formula, a 24-hour supply will be given to you in a hospital container when you leave.

What Not to Bring

Do not bring any personal linens, bath towels, face cloths, sanitary pads, routine baby clothing, or a bunch of relatives. Do not bring much money, and do not bring or wear valuables. Give any jewelry to your husband to take home. Remove heavy makeup and false eyelashes. If you wear contacts, leave them at home. Spit out your gum!

Questions You May Need to Answer When You Enter the Hospital

Many hospitals maintain complete files on expectant mothers who are due to deliver. These files are supplied by the doctors and kept in the labor suite so they will be immediately available should you come in unexpectedly or if for some reason your doctor is not immediately available. Here are the questions:

- Your name. Don't laugh; you may forget it or you may give your maiden name. It's happened.
- Your expected date of confinement (EDC).
- Your blood type and Rh factor.
- Pregnancy rank (first, second, etc.).
- Your doctor's name.
- Your pediatrician's name.
- Did your membranes rupture? When?
- Contractions—how often, how long, and where you feel them.
- Bleeding—amount and color.
- Baby movement.
- Last food—what and when.
- Disposition of contact lenses, jewelry, etc.
- False teeth or bridges. These may not need to come out, but a delivery table is no place for us to find out that they are there.
- Do you plan to nurse?
- Any known allergies—to medicine or other substances.
- Were X rays taken or ultrasound used during pregnancy, and why?
- Any medical complications or any information your doctor has advised you to give.

Remember the constant plea—if you think you are in labor, *eat nothing*. Drink fluids sparingly or not at all if you are laboring actively.

What Happens in the Hospital

It is difficult to tell you exactly what will happen in the hospital, since there are now so many different techniques of managing labor that all sorts of variables can occur. (If you have been privileged to attend classes, you already know more or less what will happen.)

Basically, first you are examined by a qualified physician or nurse to determine if you are in labor and to assess your general condition. Such examinations include temperature, pulse, respiratory rate, blood pressure, observation of contractions, fetal heart rate and regularity, evidence of bleeding or ruptured membranes. If it is confirmed that you are in labor or potentially so, or if it is determined that your membranes have truly ruptured, then you are advised to stay at the hospital. You will undoubtedly have a mini-shave around the vagina, although you can do this yourself at home, and more than likely you will have the indignity of a small enema to cleanse your lower bowel. You can do that at home, too.

After these opening ceremonies, you may go to a labor room for observation, you may go visit your family, or they may come to you. You may be monitored, sedated, have an epidural anesthetic—any number of things may happen, depending on the circumstances, the hospital, and the plans you have made with your doctor. Sooner or later you will most likely be connected to intravenous solutions, which run constantly for the remainder of your labor, delivery, and recovery period. Why these fluids? Here are some good reasons:

- Since your oral fluid intake has terminated and since you are working (that's why it is called labor), you begin to lose fluid and become dehydrated. This is particularly true in Lamaze labors, which tend to last longer and in which fluid loss through lungs (during deep breathing) is tremendous. Intravenous (IV) fluids replace the losses in all these cases.

- You also consume energy while you labor, and the sugar in your IV fluids conserves your own sugar reserves, so you don't end up burning fat. Fat is a poor fuel that produces acidosis while burning. Acidosis affects your performance in labor, but also, and more important, it can produce acidosis in your baby, depressing its respiratory centers. The use of sugar in the IV solution, however, must be carefully restricted to your immediate needs.
- Medications needed for control of labor, of pain, of blood pressure, or of any emergency can be administered through the IV and take effect at once. Such medication dosages can be meticulously controlled, and thus overdosage and delayed effects can be prevented.

There are other important reasons for giving intravenous fluids during labor, but these are the basic ones. Modern plastic needles are almost painless, can stay in place for an unlimited time, and allow you to move your arms at will with no discomfort.

Sooner or later you go to the delivery room. There, awake or asleep, you have your feet put into stirrups and, with as much dignity as possible, your bottom washed with sterile fluids and covered with drapes. Soon you and your baby will be separated. If your husband, partner, or friend is with you, fine. If not and you are awake, you may take your newborn to him—on a stretcher, that is. If you are asleep, someone will keep him posted till you can be with him. In most hospitals you may hold and cuddle your baby as soon as it is born and may hold and cuddle it again once it has been cleaned and warmed. It will be left with you and your husband from that point on, in order that bonding may proceed. Finally, you will be taken to a recovery room for an hour or two. Here specialized attendants can watch your vital signs during this critical period, observe the contractions of your uterus and sometimes massage your abdomen, assisting the contractions in their work of shrinking the uterus. They make sure your bladder, with its newfound freedom, doesn't overfill, and that you are not bleeding excessively for any reason. In some hospitals you will be returned to a private recovery room, where your family can be with you.

When your attendants are sure that you are resting quite normally, as most likely you will be, you are taken to your room. Hospital visiting hours in the maternity section are fairly standard. Exceptions are sometimes made, but under no circumstances are visitors allowed while the babies are in their mothers' rooms. Fathers are often allowed to stay longer than other visitors during the evening visiting hours. Some hospitals allow them to sleep in. This is entirely good and proper. The babies are regularly brought out and father, mother, and baby may enjoy each other. In many hospitals brothers and sisters can visit their mother and new sibling. Some variation in routine does occur, but by and large, nothing will happen to you in the hospital without your doctor's express approval, knowledge, and order.

If your hospital has a delivery unit with birthing rooms, then you may not be moved at all during the experience. That is, in modern birthing rooms, which are generally decorated somewhat like a bedroom, when delivery is imminent, the bed can be arranged for normal delivery. Then when that is accomplished, the bed is put back together and you may stay in that room until it is time to go to your postpartum quarters. Generally in this alternate birthing environment members of your family and friends can be with you while you are laboring and even delivering.

During all these procedures your doctor and all those associated with him or her and with the delivery suite hope that you are treated in this strange environment with understanding, warmth, tenderness, tact, and care. Remember, if you are in doubt about anything, ask questions—don't hesitate.

Some Questions and Some Answers

What starts labor?

A whole series of events must come into play at about the same time in order for labor to start. In the first place, the uterus cannot, regardless of what you may think, go on growing indefinitely, as there are stretch limits to the uterine wall. That is one reason multiple pregnancies deliver early. Also, the placenta begins to age very rapidly, as shown by the decrease in its production of progesterone and in its ability to transfer food and oxygen and to remove waste products from the unborn infant. The dramatic drop in progesterone is perhaps one of the major triggering factors in the onset of labor. Third, circulating through your system is oxytocin, a substance that makes your uterus contract during labor, which is made by the anterior pituitary gland. Also circulating through your system is an enzyme that deactivates oxytocin, called oxytocinase. As you approach full term, this enzyme gradually decreases in amount and allows the oxytocin to become more active. Fourth, the fetus, the infant itself, may contain the ultimate triggering mechanism for the onset of labor. There is a variety of evidence accumulating that reveals a complicated chain of events that usually ends with the release of a prostaglandin from the baby, which floods into your system. It is probably this newly discovered biological prostaglandin that finally triggers the onset of labor.

What about abnormal positions of the baby during labor?

The commonest presenting part of the baby's body during labor is the head. Usually the head is well flexed during labor, chin on chest, and the baby is lying facedown. Occasionally the head may be sideways or lying faceup. These positions can generally be adjusted by gently turning the baby's head with instruments when the time is right. More unnatural presentations do occur, however, such as the breech, or bottom, of the child

224

entering the pelvis first. Breech deliveries can be difficult and can be damaging; for this reason we are more and more frequently resorting to cesarean section for breech presentations. Some obstetricians deliver almost all breeches by cesarean section, and this has given rise to much comment in professional and media circles. There is as yet no resolution and no certain best method to deliver breeches.

There are other exceedingly abnormal presentations, such as shoulders and hands and other parts of the body; and all these are delivered by cesarean section.

What is an incompetent cervical os?

When the cervix fails to remain closed until full term and simply falls open at any time prior to term, the resultant disorder is called an incompetent cervical os. Generally it will slip open at the same time in each and every pregnancy sustained by that particular mother. The incompetence develops as a result of either general cervical weakness, cervical tearing during previous deliveries, or surgery to the cervix. Whatever the cause, the internal band of muscle and fibrous tissue that should hold the cervix closed until the full forty weeks have gone by fails at some time or another. The cervix simply falls open and the baby is expelled. This occurs generally without any labor and is purely a mechanical defect. If recognized in time, it can be corrected by sewing the cervix shut with a nylon or similar suture, much like a purse string. This string may be cut when full term is reached, or instead a cesarean section may be performed and the suture left in place to protect future pregnancies.

What is CPD?

CPD is the abbreviation for cephalo-pelvic disproportion, a situation that arises during labor when the baby's head, because of its size or its position, or the mother's pelvis, because of its architecture, hinders passage of the one through the other. Sometimes this can be predicted before the onset of labor if the maternal bony architecture is very small or has been deformed by disease or injury. Usually, however, one has to await the onset of labor to see if the disproportion between the baby's head and the mother's pelvis is such that labor cannot progress. In any event, as soon as CPD is identified and cannot safely be overcome, then delivery, of course, is by cesarean section. Some women are able to deliver one or two children normally without difficulty and all of a sudden develop CPD and have to be sectioned in this later pregnancy. Such a situation could arise from two circumstances. First, her other children may have been small—say, between five and six pounds—and the present one weigh say nine or ten pounds. Second, the labor may be such that the child's head is presenting in a very abnormal position and simply cannot negotiate the structure of its mother's pelvic canal.

I am an unwed mother and I plan to keep my child and raise it myself. What are your thoughts on this matter?

My thoughts on this matter may not be very important, since it is a social rather than a technical problem; however, here they are for what they're worth.

It is becoming much more popular for single mothers to keep their babies and raise them themselves. It is their right to do so and, with certainty, if a single mother is not delinquent in her child's care, no court in the world would take her child from her. However, it is extremely unlikely that even under the best circumstances she can provide the proper environment for raising a normal, healthy child. The chances are very good that she will come to resent the child before too long, since it will act somewhat like a millstone around her neck, preventing the development of her own personality and the continuation of her personal life.

A further fact that must be considered is that legal rights of fatherless children are questioned by many courts in the United States. The world today, particularly our country, is filled with groups crying out for their rights—women demanding their freedom, minorities vying for equal recognition. But there is no one to represent unborn babies and their rights: whether they should in fact be allowed to live or be aborted; whether they are entitled to live in a home full of warmth and understanding, with parents to take care of their emotional and physical needs. Finally, then, I would ask you to consider the rights of your child.

What is the significance of the Leboyer method of delivery?

Dr. Leboyer believes that delivery into this world is a traumatic experience—and so it is and has been since the beginning of time. We seem to be well adapted to this, however, since most of us survive without apparent significant personality damage. According to Leboyer, the whole world might improve if we could have a less traumatic experience at birth. Therefore, he has orchestrated the birth process into a quiet, orderly procedure in which the child is delivered with as little manipulation as possible and as little lighting as possible, with no attempts made to stimulate the child into crying, and with the suppression of any traumatic activity after birth. The child is laid on its mother's abdomen, stroked gently and treated compassionately. Shortly after, it is lowered into a warm bath and is encouraged to smile and react in a positive fashion.

Let me hasten to point out that most deliveries today are not conducted as they are on television and on the movie screen. We do not forcibly extract a baby and then beat its bottom in order to make it cry. This is very bad obstetrics, always has been and always will be. Most newborn children are treated gently, and if there is any degree of shock associated with the delivery or the labor, the child is treated with a gentleness and care that you would not believe. In this regard I couldn't agree more with what Dr. Leboyer preaches, and I and most other practicing obstetricians do just that. We do, however, like to see what we are doing and what is happening to the mother, so we prefer to use sufficient light. We also favor a quiet delivery room so that we can concentrate on our work, but we do like to hear the child cry on occasion after birth, particularly since we know that such crying is expanding the terminal sacs of its lungs. As I said before in regard to fads, there is basic truth in most of them, but at some point they leave reality and presuppose things that are not proved or perhaps don't exist. That's why they don't last.

Bonding

The concept of bonding and its application to obstetrics began in Case Western Reserve University's School of Medicine in Cleveland some ten years ago and since that time has received a great deal of study and interest among physicians and an equal amount of study and interest in the popular press.

Bonding begins in the uterus, where your unborn begins to recognize your voice and your touch. But it is at birth that the intensity of this relationship can soar, now that you can all see one another, feel, hear clearly, and speak softly to one another and so come to bond forever. Although this psychological fusion is deepest between mother and child, all members of the family belong in such a bond. Present-day childbirth techniques and hospital environments make bonding a great deal easier to accomplish. Thus at the time of delivery the newborn is placed where both husband and wife can touch and feel it and talk with it from the moment of birth. And in a normal, healthy situation, this close, warm contact is allowed to continue for several hours.

As with all things that are new, we have to be careful not to carry it to the extreme. The extreme would be, again, making someone feel guilty about not wanting a prolonged bonding experience at birth or, worse still, because of some abnormality in labor and delivery, about not being able to or allowed to bond. Thus from the original concept of bonding that was very highly structured and considered absolutely necessary for success, emphasis has now shifted to areas of human adaptability and to the possibility of many other fail-safe routes to attachment and, therefore, bonding.

There are many ways parents can become close and emotionally involved with their babies, and early contact is just one of them. Thus, though bonding is the *ideal* mechanism, it is not the *only* one. No one should feel hurt or a sense of shame or guilt because of being unable, for whatever reason, to do it at the moment of birth. After all, until ten years ago none of us was even aware of the concept—except mothers and babies who have forever been aware of it and have always done it instinctively.

Fascinating Facts

▷ The word *obstetric* comes from the latin word *obstare,* which is a verb meaning "to protect or stand by."

▷ In 1983 there were 2,710 women members of the American College of Obstetricians and Gynecologists. This is triple the number of members as of 1976 and represents a doubling of women's representation in the profession during that period of time. The President of the American College of Obstetricians and Gynecologists at this time (1984) is a woman—Luella Klein, M.D., of Atlanta, Georgia.

DIARY

My Ninth Month

Problems ————————————————————————

Medications ————————————————————————

————————————————————————

————————————————————————

Rate of baby movement on a scale of 1–10 ——————————

Special tests ————————————————————————

Natural childbirth classes ——————————————————

————————————————————————

What's going on in the world? ————————————————

————————————————————————

————————————————————————

What's going on in my life? ——————————————————

————————————————————————

————————————————————————

My thoughts and feelings ——————————————————

————————————————————————

————————————————————————

Doctor's appointments ——————————————————

————————————————————————

Questions To Ask

————————————————————————

————————————————————————

————————————————————————

CHAPTER TEN

MY TENTH
LUNAR MONTH

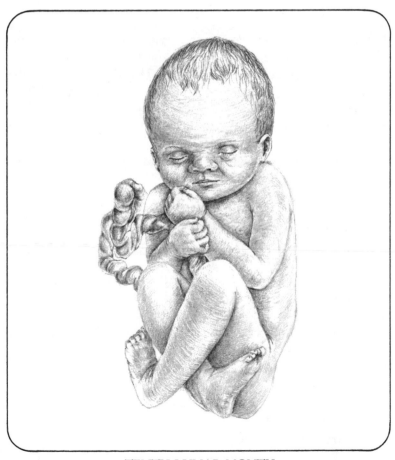

TENTH LUNAR MONTH

You're entering the tenth and last lunar month of your pregnancy—the thirty-sixth to the fortieth weeks. At the end of this period your baby is fully developed, weighing on the average 7 pounds (3150 grams) and measuring about 20 inches (52 cms) in length. The downy hair (lanugo) that covered baby's skin has now almost disappeared, but the waxy white vernix caseosa persists. Scalp hair is growing well, fingernails and toenails are about ready for clipping, and you're about ready to call it all off.

Although the average birth weight at full term is about 7 pounds, there is a great deal of individual variation, the usual range being from 5.5 to 10 pounds. Anything below that is called premature, although, as you already know, it may not be, and anything above that is considered postmature and a real drag. The largest newborn baby recorded in all known literature weighed 26 pounds net, but be consoled: It is truly exceptional for a baby to weigh over 13 pounds at birth. Again, you already know that the birth weight of a newborn child is a function of a combination of factors—its genetic or inherited background, the total duration of the pregnancy, the diet that carried you through pregnancy, and certain complicating factors, such as diabetes, which may greatly affect the size of a baby. Remember, although you are technically due at the end of this month, in a normal pregnancy you are not overdue for two more weeks.

Anesthesia and Analgesia

Strangely enough, most articles written about pain relief in obstetrics and most of the research done in this area have been the product of men's labor. We've talked about that. Also, it was a man who first insisted that women be allowed pain relief during labor and first introduced it to the birthing rooms— although Queen Victoria gave ether a mighty imperial boost when she insisted upon having it at her disposal at the time of the delivery of her son Edward, in later life to become Edward the Peacemaker, the great British monarch whose wit and wisdom seemed blunted not at all by her acceptance of this powerful pain relieving agent! At any rate, none of these male physicians, including this one, ever has had or ever will have the fortune or misfortune to experience childbearing and its pain or lack of it. Also let me point out that we didn't introduce pain relief against our patients' will or to take advantage of them in whatever way while they were in a drug-induced trance. The church and many laymen said we did—but we didn't. We did it for our patients. And thus now pain relief during labor and delivery is an integral part and a most important aspect of modern obstetrics. It consists of more than providing personal comfort to the mother; it is an absolute and a necessary part of *good* obstetrical practice. Thoughtfully chosen analgesia can improve labor, and proper anesthesia permits difficult deliveries to be accomplished with safety—and comfort.

Before proceeding further, let us define some terms.

- *Analgesia* is really stage one of a general anesthetic. At this point memory is suspended and there are varying degrees of insensitivity to pain or lack of perception of pain. Yet there is sufficient consciousness to allow protective reflexes to function, for instance, swallowing and closing of the vocal cords can be continued.

235

- *Anesthesia* represents full loss of sensation. General anesthesia not only implies loss of sensation, but it also provides loss of consciousness, motor power, and reflex activity. Local or regional anesthesia produces loss of pain sensation and motor activity by blocking sensory impulses in a given region of the body. There are many forms of regional anesthesia; in obstetrics this includes large or major blocks, such as a spinal or an epidural block, both of which are given in the lower back and are very effective, and lesser blocks, such as local infiltrations in the perineum and into the cervical or para-cervical area. Either general or regional anesthesia can provide suitable conditions for most normal and operative obstetrical procedures.

Now then, anyone who has ever been on either end of the delivery table and who is not a fanatic agrees that some parts of labor and delivery are painful. We've been over that, too. The amount of pain felt varies with:

- *The individual personal pain threshold.* It takes more pain to make some of us *feel* pain.
- *Fear.* A painful experience that is feared is doubly, triply, or infinitely more painful. Therefore, healthy preparation for childbirth helps dispel fear and so reduces pain. This is one of the greatest contributions of prepared-childbirth classes. Every expectant mother should attend such a class, at least during her first pregnancy. Childbirth education, provided properly, results in less need for pharmacological or drug pain relief. However, you should not be made to feel guilty or ashamed if you choose to utilize an acceptable mode of pharmacological pain relief as labor progresses. This has been mentioned earlier in our discussions on prepared childbirth and deserves mention again.
- *Abnormal labors.* When an abnormal presentation occurs—a breech or a badly extended head or a tight fit—any of these

236

labors and many others may be long, arduous, and painful, and a delivery without help may produce unbearable suffering.

General Principles of Obstetrical Pain Relief

Significant discomfort in the early stages of pregnancy is usually managed by the use of a variety of drugs. Most generally these drugs include barbiturates, narcotics, tranquilizers, and scopolamine or atropine, generally used in a variety of combinations. In past years they were used together to produce what was known as twilight sleep. The dosages at that time were much greater than they are today and fell into disfavor when more and more women wished or agreed to participate actively in their labor and delivery. The use of these agents, however, was characterized by a rather wide safety margin insofar as the mother and the fetus were concerned and generally were well handled by both. Today some or all of these agents are still used in the very early stages of labor and then followed, if possible, by a regional anesthetic, either an epidural or a spinal. If deeper anesthesia is needed and regional anesthesia cannot be given, for whatever reason, then a balanced inhalation anesthetic is used.

General Anesthesia

Balanced general anesthesia consists of the use of intravenous barbiturates to induce the anesthesia, accompanied by inhalation of nitrous oxide and oxygen to maintain unconsciousness. The addition of intravenous succinylcholine—a muscle paralyzer—produces deep enough anesthesia and relaxation so that even a very difficult cesarean section can be performed quite readily, and certainly any operative vaginal procedure can also be accomplished. The advantage of general versus conduction anesthesia is that it can be given by nurse anesthetists, who in many obstetrical units are readily available, while physician anesthesiologists may not be.

Besides the general availability of inhalation anesthesia, another advantage is that it displays a wide margin of safety in terms of transfer of the anesthetic agents across the placenta and, therefore, respiratory depression of the newborn infant. But there is no question that anesthetic agents do have a certain amount of depressant effect upon the newborn, particularly if the anesthesia has gone on for a long time.

Finally, inhalation anesthesia tends to induce vomiting. This is not a problem for patients who are well prepared for anesthesia, but many laboring mothers are not well prepared and have food in the stomach when they come to deliver. This is one of the reasons we caution you not to eat if you even *think* you are in labor. Even if you haven't eaten recently, gastric emptying time is delayed in early labor, and thus food tends to stay in the stomach for many hours after it has been eaten.

Regional Anesthesia

There are four types:

1. *Spinal block.* This procedure involves placing a needle within the membranes that surround the spinal nerve cord, extracting a small amount of the enclosed spinal fluid, and replacing it with anesthesia agents. This produces almost instantaneous numbness and motor paralysis from that point in the spinal canal downward. Sometimes the same reaction extends higher into the spinal canal, depending upon the type of agent used. The advantage of a spinal block is that it produces instantaneous pain relief virtually all the time, and it has no effect upon the fetus whatsoever, providing the mother's blood pressure is kept at acceptable levels.

There is a tendency for the blood pressure to fall in all block anesthetics. The disadvantage of a spinal anesthetic is that the effective duration is short—usually the maximum is 2 hours; moreover, a spinal headache that may last for several days or even weeks following spinal anesthesia is a complication in 2 percent of patients.

2. *Epidural block or lumbar epidural block.* Another form of regional anesthesia producing pain relief and some degree of motor loss, this is given in a small area just outside the membranes that coat the spinal nerve—the epidural space. Usually a tiny catheter is inserted into this area, and the anesthetic is administered and readministered through it for as long as it's necessary to complete labor and delivery. One of its advantages, therefore, is that it can be given relatively early in labor and continued throughout the remainder of labor and delivery. Another real advantage is that it's not followed by a headache. It is generally safe and well tolerated by a laboring mother, and it allows her to participate to a distinct degree in the birthing process and to watch her delivery and bond with her baby afterward. The disadvantages of lumbar blocks are few. One major problem is that an anesthesiologist or obstetrician must administer it. Although in many obstetrical units the nurse anesthetist can follow the progress of a block once it has been administered by a physician, it still must be physician-placed.

Very seldom are there any fetal effects from an epidural anesthetic. One temporary problem is a reaction to the anesthetic agent used. Some of the medication always gets into the maternal circulation and, therefore, the fetal circulation, where it is known to concentrate. This can affect the infant's heart rate, and under such circumstances delivery is postponed until the effect wears off. This event, incidentally, can be followed quite readily in a monitored labor. Also, as with spinal anesthetics, there is a tendency for hypotension or low blood pressure to follow epidural anesthetic administration. This must be carefully watched for and treated properly by correct positioning of the laboring mother and adjustment of her fluid and medicine intake to keep her blood pressure stable.

Occasionally epidural anesthesia retards labor, and so it must be augmented. On the other hand, however, epidural anesthesia sometimes accelerates the progress of labor. All in all, this particular form of regional anesthesia is probably the most popular type of obstetrical pain relief in use today.

3. *Pudendal block.* This is a local block given into the perineum and areas that surround the vagina and cervix. It is administered by the obstetrician just prior to delivery and gives adequate local anesthesia for the use of outlet forceps and performance of an episiotomy. It is of no value in any form of operative intervention. It has practically no effect on the infant unless large amounts of the local agent somehow get into the maternal circulation.

4. *Paracervical block.* This technique is also very local. As the name indicates, local anesthesia agents are injected on either side of the cervix to produce, again, local blocks of pain conduction. Its disadvantages are almost identical to those of the pudendal variety, although it is more likely to produce temporary depression of the fetal heart rate, since more of it is likely to get into the maternal circulation.

These, then, represent the common agents used in obstetrics to produce analgesia and anesthesia during labor and delivery, along with their good and bad points. It is to be hoped that long before you go into labor you have discussed with your doctor what type of pain relief you wish, if any, and he or she has pointed out any peculiarities of your own particular pregnancy that might make the choice of one over the other form of anesthesia more rational. Undoubtedly this subject will come up several times during the course of your prenatal visits.

Anesthesia for Cesarean Section

Either regional or general anesthesia may be used for a cesarean-section delivery. Many times an epidural anesthetic is in place and functioning when the decision is made to do a cesarean section, and so it may simply be continued. However, there are times when regional anesthesia is not the choice, and a general anesthetic is substituted.

A regional anesthetic would be favored if the patient to be operated upon has a full stomach, has a respiratory infection or respiratory disease, or some other anticipated airway difficulty. On the other hand, a general anesthetic is to be preferred if a rapid delivery is necessary, such as in instances in which relaxation of a tetanically contracted uterus is needed, or when there is excessive maternal bleeding or a clotting disorder, a systemic infection, or a preexisting neurological disorder—all these and other conditions call for general anesthesia.

So in operative obstetrics there is room for and a need for both types of anesthesia. And again, your doctor will surely discuss the advantages and the disadvantages of both of them in your case, and you will use the one most suitable to your needs.

Labor

Labor is the forceful expulsion of a baby and its afterbirth from the uterus through the vagina. It usually begins within a few

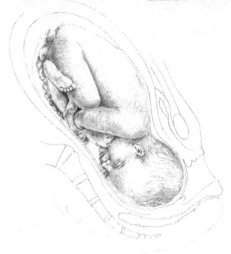

1. DELIVERY CONTRACTIONS

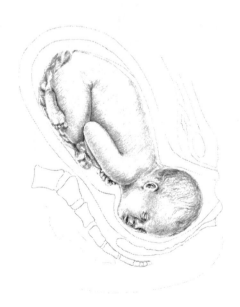

2. DILATION OF CERVIX

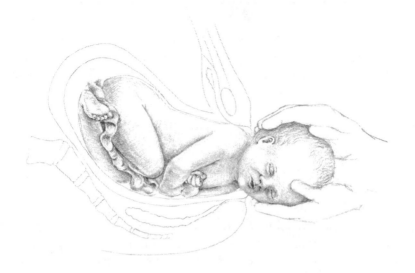

3. DELIVERY OF HEAD

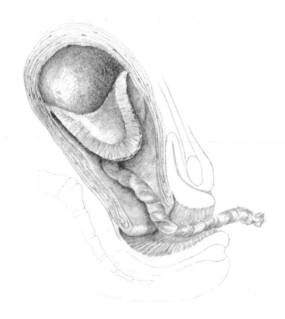

4. DELIVERY OF PLACENTA

weeks on either side of day 265, and in the first pregnancy usually lasts about 12 hours; in subsequent pregnancies, 6 to 8 hours. There are wide variations, however, within all these limits.

False Labor

During the last few weeks of pregnancy the uterus is contracting with considerable vigor, and it is not unusual for some of the contractions to be moderately painful. If, as occasionally happens, these episodes become regular and painful, you then have false labor. The contraction pattern in false labor may be very regular, that is, you may have contractions at 5-minute intervals, lasting about half a minute, and this may go on for many hours. But there are several differences between false and true labor.

- False labor goes nowhere. No matter how long it continues, there is no dilation of the cervix. Only true labor accomplishes this.
- Although the contractions may be regular and uncomfortable, generally the interval between them remains about the same no matter how long the pains last. Thus if at the end of 8 hours the interval is still 8 minutes, it is most likely false labor.
- The contractions of false labor will eventually disappear or can be made to disappear with mild sedatives or pain medication.

Despite all this, it is sometimes difficult to tell false from true labor, and you must consult your doctor if you are in doubt. Even he or she may not be sure, and occasionally if you exhibit these contractions, your doctor will admit you to the hospital and watch you carefully in order to determine exactly what is going on.

True Labor

True labor usually begins with the same sort of menstruallike cramps that herald the onset of a period, often beginning in your lower back and swinging around into your lower abdomen. Frequently such cramps are as much as half an hour apart, but they soon get closer, longer, and harder. Your doctor will probably want you to call him or her when the contractions are about 8 to 10 minutes apart.

In rare instances labor begins suddenly, with pains that are very close together and produce much discomfort. Under these circumstances you should call as soon as you are sure what is what. Also, labor may begin with or be preceded by a discharge of bloody mucus, called show. You need not call your doctor if show appears, since active labor may be hours away, but if you have any heavy bleeding from the vagina, call immediately.

Occasionally the membranes rupture before labor begins or during early labor. Fluid gushes from the vagina or trickles constantly and uncontrollably. When you feel that your membranes have ruptured, you should report it to your doctor and put down the pizza. Very, very rarely a tragic accident may happen when the membranes rupture. If the baby is not sitting well in the pelvis or is in an abnormal position, the umbilical cord may prolapse when the membranes rupture. Should that occur—and again, it is exceedingly rare—hopefully enough cord will come down that you can feel it protruding from your vagina. In that event, feel to be sure that it is pulsating; as long as it is pulsating, your baby will be fine. Even if you cannot be sure about pulsations, you must lie down immediately and put several pillows under your bottom to keep baby's presenting part from dropping into the pelvis. Your head, upper body, and abdomen should be considerably below your pelvis and lower extremities. Someone else must call an ambulance and get you to a hospital in that same position, maintaining constant vigilance to be sure that the cord is continuing to pulsate. Again, this is a most unusual happenstance, but quick treatment can prevent a catastrophe.

Stages of Labor

The expulsion of your child into the world by labor is divided into three stages. The purpose of labor, of course, is to dilate the cervix completely, push the presenting part—usually the head—through the pelvis, and deliver the baby out to the world: probably the shortest and most dangerous trip your child will ever take.

In the *first* stage of labor, the cervix dilates completely. Labor usually begins with the cervix somewhere between 1 to 3 centimeters (½–1 inch) dilated. Complete dilation—10 centimeters—usually requires some 8 to 10 hours in the first pregnancy, often considerably less in subsequent pregnancies. During this time the presenting part, usually the head, is most likely descending into and through the pelvic canal. Dilation of the cervix is accomplished in effect by reduction of the volume in the uterine cavity. The uterine contractions you felt throughout most of your pregnancy might be likened to flexing your arm, thus tightening the muscles and then letting the arm straighten again and relaxing the whole muscle. Now that labor has begun, the contractions change in a very significant way. Each time the muscles tighten, they grow a little shorter; comparing it to your arm again, each time you flex the muscle, your elbow will bend a little more, until finally your hand is touching your shoulder. Thus, in the uterine cavity, as the muscle fibers grow shorter, the capacity of the uterus to contain your baby diminishes and so it pushes against the cervix to find a way out. The cervix, being properly prepared, dilates to provide that way out.

During the first stage of labor there is no advantage to

voluntary pushing or bearing down, nor should you feel any desire to do so. Such muscular activity would only exhaust you, and you cannot push a baby through an unopened cervix any more than you can push yourself through an unopened door. You are generally receiving fluids intravenously at this time. Most likely a monitor is attached to your abdomen. You may have been given some medication for pain relief. If you are going to have an epidural anesthetic, it is customarily administered when dilation has reached 3 to 4 centimeters (2 inches), but this may be delayed if your labor is very slow, if the head is not well into the pelvis, or if you have no particular desire for pain relief at this time. If you are practicing natural childbirth, during the first stage of labor all attempts are directed to achieving the utmost in relaxation and the conversion of pain sensation to other sensations.

In the *second* stage of labor, the cervix is completely dilated and the baby needs to be pushed out into the world. This may take a minute or it may take several hours. Generally, the more babies you have, the quicker it takes place. If you have received no anesthesia, you will experience an intense urge to bear down, such as you would during a bowel movement. It is at this time that the voluntary muscular system comes into play, and actively pushing and bearing down with your abdominal muscles can be of great assistance.

If you have had an epidural anesthetic, you will have no feeling whatsoever at this time. The contractions of the uterus as it continually decreases in size continue to force the baby through the pelvic canal and out into your doctor's waiting hands. In order to shorten the second stage, particularly if there is an abnormal presentation of the head, it may be necessary to use forceps to turn the head or simply to ease it over the entrance of the vagina. Regardless of what you may have heard, such forceps applications are very safe. Your doctor will also most likely perform an episiotomy (see p. 248) during the final phase of the second stage. Your baby, if it is well, will be given to you on your tummy so that bonding may begin.

The *third* stage of labor represents the expulsion of the placenta. It can occur very abruptly after delivery of the child or may require many minutes and some assistance. A number of doctors are now removing the placenta manually after the delivery, but many still wait for the natural separation to occur and the placenta to slip out by itself. There is nothing you can do to aid in this stage of labor. You are probably not even thinking about it as you cuddle your newborn child. Very frequently before the placenta delivers, routine samples of blood are taken from the umbilical cord, to be sent to the laboratory to determine the baby's blood type and whether any significant antibodies are present, and to do other blood tests if indicated. For instance, if the baby was depressed for any reason at birth, the doctor would probably want to get blood oxygen and carbon dioxide saturation as well as blood pH determinations to evaluate the degree of depression.

Sooner or later the placenta is delivered, and that part is finished. Your doctor then explores the birth canal for any retained tissue or membranes or evidence of a tear, and if all is well, he sews up your episiotomy and his work is completed. Yours, however, is just beginning. Meanwhile your baby is cleaned and its Apgar (see Glossary) score taken to determine its degree of stability. Now it is placed again in your arms for you and your husband to admire; if your husband is not with you in the delivery room, you are then wheeled out to show the baby to your husband and family.

Again this warning: If you think you are in labor, or if your membranes have ruptured, *do not eat or drink* anything from that moment on. Call your doctor for further instructions.

Induction of Labor

To induce labor is to purposely set in motion the process of labor at a selected time preceding the onset of natural labor. There are two types of induced labor: indicated and elective. An indicated induction is undertaken when there is some condition of the mother or her unborn child (or both) that makes early delivery necessary. Severe hypertension of pregnancy or a positive contraction stress test might be considered typical reasons for an indicated induction. This procedure must sometimes be attempted as much as a month before the baby is due, and because things are not ready inside, it is often difficult and dangerous. However, the risks of waiting longer are even greater. Indicated inductions used to be called forced labor.

An elective induction presupposes that the pregnancy is perfectly normal, that the mother is at full term and her baby a good size, and that all conditions are favorable for a regular delivery. This, then, is a convenience type of delivery. It makes it easier for the mother to make her arrangements at home, for her to get to the hospital in comfort—especially if she labors rapidly—and to be certain that the hospital and delivery room crew are at full strength. Since these deliveries are for the convenience of the mother, her family, and the doctor, it is extremely important that there be no greater risk incurred than if the labor were to occur naturally.

In well-documented studies of thousands upon thousands of controlled elective inductions of labor, it has been shown beyond doubt that the intelligent induction of labor by a skilled practitioner carries with it less risk to both mother and child than does spontaneous labor. Emphasis, however, must be placed upon the facts that the mother must be selected carefully for this procedure and the doctor must be skilled in the induction of labor.

Sometimes, when labor is to be induced, you are asked to

come to the hospital the night before. You receive the usual amenities—shave and enema plus, if you are lucky, a sedative. Early the next morning an intravenous is inserted and oxytocin slowly pumped in. Your contractions and your baby are monitored as in normal labor, and so it goes.

Episiotomy

We have seen that during the second stage of labor your child is pushed out into the world. Although the vagina is capable of a great deal of stretching, the muscles and skin that make it up can and do tear and sustain damage at the time of delivery. Most often during your first delivery and most of those that follow, it is common for your doctor to do an episiotomy, that is, make an incision into the muscles and skin of the vagina and the skin on the outside as well, in order to prevent a tear. Thus, after your child and its placenta are delivered, this incision is a clean, straight wound that is easy to repair, whereas a tear would be jagged and rough and difficult to repair decently. Occasionally an episiotomy is not necessary because tissues stretch satisfactorily or have already been stretched by a previous delivery.

Although your episiotomy may cause you some discomfort after you deliver, it heals much better than a tear and gives you much better support for later years. Most episiotomies are repaired with suture material that dissolves and does not have to be removed after delivery. One of the most common questions a doctor is asked after delivery is: "How many stitches were used to repair my episiotomy?" This is a difficult question to answer, for many of our suture techniques resemble hemstitching, that is, we use one continuous suture throughout most or all of the episiotomy, taking small stitches just as you would in hemming a skirt. This is much better than basting the incision or taking a couple of big stitches. (A suture, then, may consist of a single separate stitch or a number of running stitches.)

Therefore, the answer to that question is meaningless. Believe me, it is better to have a hundred small stitches than two great big grabbers.

Lately the episiotomy, as with so many other important things, has fallen victim to the frantic race among some of the avant-garde and cultists to get motherhood back to nature before things get too good. Many women who do not receive interventions such as a deep and proper episiotomy tend to develop several specific disorders from the resultant muscle and skin damage. The rectum and the bladder tend to push through the damaged muscle support and bulge into the vagina, causing conditions known as rectocele (from the rectum) and cystocele (from the bladder), which require surgical intervention somewhere along the line. Relaxation of the vagina can also lead to a loss of sexual sensation. This loss of sexual sensation is felt (or not felt) by both partners. The extremists of the "natural" movement ignore this problem and state that psychogenic stimulation outside the vagina compensates for the loss of vaginal sensation, which is exactly the same as saying smelling ice cream is as good as eating it. Although the back-to-nature movement is a well-intended, highly motivated trend toward a certain psychological end point through education and training, the end point of its adherents, so far as episiotomies are concerned, remains obscure.

Forceps

Although you remember I said that forceps were introduced by a doctor in the last century and incidentally revolutionized obstetrics, that is probably not correct. At least not entirely correct. It is altogether likely that forceps of a sort were invented in ancient times and ancient cultures but that the techniques were lost for centuries thereafter. Forceps of a modern type are still used to extract babies mechanically from their mothers. Forceps deliveries are the so-called instrument deliveries. When they were first used, forceps were reserved for the most difficult obstructed labors, and the results, as might be imagined, were not too good. Presently forceps are used primarily to shorten the second stage of labor and the prolonged pounding of the baby's head against the mother's tissues. The use of forceps in this situation is not dangerous; it does not harm either mother or child in any known way.

Occasionally forceps have to be used to turn a baby that is lying abnormally in its mother's pelvis and has thus caused progress in labor to cease. Such forceps deliveries are considerably more difficult to execute, but the danger to mother and baby is still not great. The situations that occasioned the very damaging and drastic forceps deliveries of older days are now simply resolved by cesarean section.

Another type of instrument delivery is used in many areas of this country and abroad. It is called a vacuum extractor and, pardon the comparison, works something like a plumber's helper! A rubber or plastic cup is applied to the infant's head, and a suction device produces a vacuum between the head and the extractor. The physician then uses this to put gentle traction on the child's head and turn and deliver it through the pelvis. The advocates of this device say that it is less likely to damage the child or the mother's small parts, and they certainly have a good argument. The instrument will probably be used increasingly to assist in the termination of the second stage of labor.

Overdue?

The last time we talked about being overdue, you had just missed a period; now you are missing a baby! Although you have been told that you are not overdue until you have gone at least two weeks beyond the expected date of delivery, as far as you are concerned, you were overdue at midnight yesterday. Your family and in-laws and all your friends feel the same way and very frequently express this conviction. But they are wrong.

In a normal, healthy pregnancy the onset of labor may occur anywhere within two weeks before or two weeks after the expected day of confinement. And that is a fact.

One of the problems we face in dating a pregnancy is that we are not always certain of the exact duration of the pregnancy, and even the two people involved are not often absolutely certain when the fruitful union took place. The information that we have to assess to determine the correct dates includes when contraception ceased, the date of the last menstrual period, the determination of pregnancy duration on your first pelvic examination, the appearance of an audible heartbeat, and the rate of uterine growth as pregnancy advances. Two specific tests that may be of great help are the pregnancy test, which, if done very early in pregnancy, is a really good clue to pregnancy duration, and, of course, an ultrasound, which is probably the greatest help of all. (Turn to Appendix to learn how ultrasound can determine pregnancy duration.)

Should the pregnancy last beyond forty-two weeks, it becomes a different problem entirely. It is now called a postmature or a postdate pregnancy, and it is watched very closely indeed by obstetricians. Five percent of all pregnancies end up in this category. Remember that the placenta reaches its maximum function at thirty-seven weeks and is thereafter gradually deteriorating. What we are looking for in most postdate pregnancies is the maintenance of placental function and, therefore, fetal nourishment and oxygenation.

Around the forty-second week of a confirmed pregnancy, most often your obstetrician will induce labor, providing the cervix is favorable for induction (see elective induction, p. 247). If, however, the condition of the cervix is not favorable, then all or some of the tests of fetal well-being are brought into play: nonstress test, contraction stress test, biophysical profile, amniocentesis, blood hormone levels, and so forth (see Appendix). If these show any evidence of fetal stress and the cervix is still unfavorable, delivery by cesarean section will probably be resorted to. If the tests show no fetal stress or distress, then the pregnancy will probably be allowed to continue for another week or two until the cervix becomes favorable. During this time, tests for fetal well-being are continued, and you will probably be asked by your obstetrician to score fetal movement on a daily basis yourself. By following these plans in managing the postdate pregnancy in recent years, the incidence of fetal damage and fetal death has gradually been whittled down. Remember that there are wide variations in all these things, and your obstetrician may not follow my plan exactly as it has been outlined.

Room and Bored

In those lazy hazy days of the recent past, women used to luxuriate in the hospital for ten days or so, even after the most uneventful delivery! Clean sheets, twice-daily back rubs, good food and no dishes to wash, baby away somewhere in a distant nursery getting fed, washed, changed, and spoiled by some nurse! It was a piece of cake. Seems foolish for you to have taken up arms against treatment like that, doesn't it?

Well, ten days in the hospital would bankrupt most young families today—and besides, it wasn't all as good as it sounds. Those mothers were kept in bed too long and suffered a multitude of problems because of it, some of them very serious. Anyway, those days are gone forever, and the average postpartum stay is now about two days or, in the case of a section, about four.

What goes on in those few days? Well, it's not as boring as you might think, and, if your baby is rooming in, a whole lot goes on. Dad is with you part of the time and your baby all the time. Even if you do not have rooming in, it is still a pretty busy place. Visitors will be in to see you, depending upon your hospital's regulations. It is good to abide by these regulations since they are meant to protect you and your baby, and sometimes there can be too many good things and good visitors! Visitors often forget their social and their smoking manners— and while we're on that subject, if you are sharing your room with another mother who doesn't smoke, please be considerate of her. By now you were supposed to have quit anyway!

Hospital schedules are funny, to say the least, and may seem to be arranged for doctors' and nurses' convenience—and that may be partly true. So you may be getting up when you used to go to bed and eating your evening meal during the soaps! Incidentally, some hospitals give mom and dad a champagne dinner the first night after delivery. Even if your hospital does not, they probably wouldn't mind if somebody brought this celebration to you. Like Dad.

Here are some things to observe about your own bodily functions during these lying-in days.

- You have a bloody vaginal discharge no matter how you delivered. This discharge is called lochia. It may be heavier than a period at first but rapidly diminishes over the next few days. Sanitary pads must be worn—you cannot use a tampon until someone says you can, which will be awhile. Lochia comes from the uterus, mainly the placental site, and as the uterus shrinks to normal size over the next two weeks, the bleeding decreases. It may not stop completely until many weeks have gone by.
- You may have been catheterized to remove urine from your bladder. This may have been done during labor and again at delivery. Because of this and the stresses put on your bladder during labor and delivery, it is not uncommon to have mild discomfort on voiding. Sometimes the bladder is temporarily paralyzed, and an in-dwelling catheter must be inserted and left for a day or perhaps even longer. All these unusual things make the bladder more likely to get infected (cystitis). It is important to drink lots of fluids and to urinate frequently. Report any signs of burning and/or urgent urination.

- Pains of various kinds may beset you.

"Afterpains" are like labor contractions, and they represent the same type of uterine muscular activity. They usually last several days, are more common after the first pregnancy, and are harder while you are nursing. Suckling is nature's way of making your uterus come down in size, but it is somewhat painful. At times, particularly in the second or third pregnancy, afterpains can be real attention getters, but soon are gone.

Your episiotomy is in a very sensitive place—between the vagina and rectum—and can cause you some discomfort as you move about. Speaking of moving, you may hope that your bowels do not move again, ever! But they will, and all will stay together. In some hospitals you can take a sitz bath several times each day, and this gives great local relief. Continue to do it at home. Your doctor has probably ordered creams or other medications that will also give you area relief. No matter what is done— or not done—the discomfort gradually leaves completely, although for many months the episiotomy site may throb uncomfortably during the first few days of each period.

Breast discomfort arrives about the time you are ready to go home. Your breasts become very congested, but not with milk. That comes in a day or so after the congestion. Whether or not nursing is your goal, support your breasts with a good bra, but not tightly, and use local heat or cold—whatever feels best. Milk appears shortly after the congestion. Breast infections are unusual and do not appear until later. The symptoms are fever, local redness, and pain. This is a doctor situation.

As a result of the bearing down required of you and because of the local rectal dilation, hemorrhoids are not unusual. As in the earlier instructions on hemorrhoid care, avoid straining when you move your bowels, be

254

sure you are getting bulk and a stool softener in your diet, and, if necessary, ask for local medications for pain relief. Generally speaking, your bowel function should return promptly after delivery, unless elimination has always been a problem for you. In such a case, you should already have a bowel program.

Blues

We have already talked about "baby blues," and you know that it can happen to you—no matter how happy you are and how well things seem to be going. Even in your most joyous moments you may burst out crying. But don't despair; it is transient and will soon be gone.

Hygiene

Your personal hygiene need not change much after a vaginal delivery, except that you cannot wear tampons (I don't think you would want to anyway) and you cannot douche. Otherwise you may shower and wash your hair and may also tub bathe. Sometimes, as we already noted, sitting in the tub a spell brings considerable relief to weary, painful areas. Most hospitals provide facilities to do these cleansing things, and you will feel better for it.

After a Section

You are now both postoperative and postpartum. You are likely to recover a little more slowly after a section, and the feelings are different than after a vaginal delivery. The first day you probably stay in bed and have an in-dwelling bladder catheter. You may be fed intravenously. There is more discomfort at the operative site, and you are given somewhat stronger pain relief. Generally, by the second day your catheter has been removed and you are encouraged to get up (with help) and move about. Oral feedings are started, and you progress to a full diet as rapidly as you can tolerate hospital food. Probably the next two days are made memorable to you by copious gas, which collects in your colon and thunderously awaits your recovering ability to expel it. This usually happens during visiting hours! At any rate, you will be glad to see and hear the last of it. Sometimes that departure requires an enema. But once your bowels have responded, you are ready to hit the trail. At home you require more rest and help than you would following a vaginal delivery. Recovery from abdominal surgery such as a cesarean section is much more rapid and uneventful than it used to be. But you must pace yourself.

Some Things to Note About Your Hospital Stay

- Your doctor or an associate or a nurse practitioner will see you almost every day. Should you have a pediatrician, he or she will also see you daily. It may be hard to know what questions to ask which, but don't hesitate to ask anything of anyone. This is particularly true about topics such as nursing and, should you have a son, circumcision.
- Speaking of circumcision, the operation is not done routinely anymore. If you want it done or if your pediatrician recommends it, you must sign a consent form, and one of your doctors will do it before you leave. Don't neglect to discuss this.
- Rh vaccination. If you are Rh negative be sure that your vaccination program is carried out if necessary. This is almost never overlooked in any hospital setting, but it is worth double checking.
- Rubella. If you are not already immune to German measles, now is a good time to be vaccinated. All you have to do is keep from getting pregnant for the next sixty days! You've survived greater challenges than that.

Homecoming

The chocolates are gone, the roses are wilted, your elbows are raw from hospital sheets, you are tired of being awakened to see if you are asleep, you are tired of having lunch at breakfast-time, you can now sit down without swearing—and so it's homeward bound. Because going home with your new baby represents a most critical time in your married life, let's begin your homecoming instructions with a bit of philosophy concerning love, marriage, and sharing.

It is very important in marriage, as in all things, to put first things first. Unfortunately, because of a repeated error in our cultural pattern, and because of the impact of advertising in women's magazines, on television, and in the press, we tend to get the order of importance of things in marriage reversed. Daily we are reminded that our children—their bonding, their education, health and security—come first. Next comes a clean kitchen and the proper selection of detergents and coffee. After all this comes social, school, religious, and cultural responsibilities, including the PTA, the Little League, the sale of Girl Scout cookies, and the ERA. After that comes your makeup, the length of your hem, and the state of your cooking. And last, unless I've forgotten something else of greater importance, your husband and your relationship with him.

The truth, of course, is that this order should be reversed. The most important single thing in your life, other than your own identity, self-love, and growth as an individual, is your husband and your relationship with him both socially and sexually, and not necessarily in that order. If your relationship with him doesn't come first, nothing else, in the long run, will be meaningful and satisfactory for either of you. We are apparently the sexiest unwed society going. But once we are married, it all seems to cease. Whoever saw a husband and wife kiss on a TV commercial? Really kiss? But this is life, not TV, so don't just keep your husband around for sentimental reasons. Cleave to him and rap with him! End of lecture.

When you come home from the hospital, remember that this is a very critical time. I hope your doctor has impressed this upon you. To begin with, you are not as strong as you thought you were when you left the hospital, and you have a new, 24-hour, demanding, loving responsibility and no nurse to hand it back to after feeding time. And, for that matter, no nurse to bring food to you or to make your bed.

Moreover, your husband may not easily adjust to sharing you and your love with this new responsibility, particularly if it is the firstborn. You must understand that he loves you and that he loves the baby, but he is perhaps jealous of his position in your loving order. I repeat: Your husband comes first; baby comes second.

Equally important, you may be somewhat depressed because of the "baby blues." Although this is usually a mild complaint, it is a contributing factor at this uncertain time.

Then, as a final blow, you may have friends or relatives ever-present around you, suggesting, interfering, confusing you. They are usually as pleasant and helpful as sand in your bathing suit but not nearly as easy to get rid of. You may soon feel that *you* had an operation and *they* had a baby.

In view of all these factors, a good plan for the early days at home would be as follows:

Unless you dwell in a mansion and are accustomed to servants, don't have anybody living in except your husband. Get your help from him. You may need extra day help with cleaning, shopping, and so on, but have as little as possible. Your mother or his mother may wish to come and help, and if they do and it is necessary, then as soon as possible make it on your own. Don't have visitors unless you want them. Get your advice from your doctor. As soon as you are able, step out with your husband without your baby and keep your private life going. You are not a slave, and it was never intended that you spend the rest of your days and nights cooped up in a house or an apartment doing the same dull things over and over again. That leads to "cabin fever," and cabin fever leads to trouble. Remember that!

Make your baby feel secure and loved when you are together, but learn to leave it with others for short periods of time. After all, at eighteen or so—if you're lucky—this loving child is going to shake your hand, say "Thanks a lot for everything," and leave. If you have made a pattern of devoting your entire life to that child, you will find yourself with thirty or forty years left over to share with no one. This is good advice. Your family and relatives may not agree—but take a close look at their experience.

Activities

It is difficult to say exactly how active any individual mother can be when she gets home from the hospital. There is a tremendous variation in energy levels. You probably find that you tire more easily than you might expect, and you must key your activities to this fact. Since you are up at night for some weeks to come, try to establish an afternoon sleep period each day. If you continually push yourself too hard, you only delay your complete recovery.

You may go outside and you may go up stairs whenever you wish. If you are willing to face traffic, there is no reason you cannot go for an automobile ride whenever you want. You may drive the car yourself when you feel steady enough. Buckle up everybody.

Although your stomach muscles and skin have been stretched greatly by pregnancy and are loose and flabby, they are yours to keep. For the sake of your posture, your back, and your self-esteem, you need to get these muscles toned again as soon as you can. You may begin exercising at any time, even while you are still in the hospital, and even if you have had a cesarean section. The trouble is—and you soon find this out—there is very little time and energy left over for formal exercises. But ask the physical therapist in the hospital to demonstrate a series of exercises. The rest is up to you.

The best solution to the exercise problem is to become involved in some outdoor sport activity, weather permitting. You may choose swimming, tennis, or golf, all of which are ready for you as soon as you are ready for them. Bicycling and horseback riding are ready for you whenever your bottom is ready. More aggressive activities, such as water skiing, should be delayed three or four weeks, but the key is to *get out* and *get active* in something that is interesting and exercise those flabby muscles. Aerobics provide an excellent way to get started in this program.

Hygiene

As you have seen, hospital routines allow you to shower, bathe, and wash your hair anytime you wish. Moreover, you are encouraged to take sitz baths to help heal your episiotomy. When you get home, instead of taking a sitz bath, just go ahead and take a full tub bath, which is both cleansing and healing. You may also, of course, shower and shampoo. But if you shower rather than bathe, be sure your perineum, the area of your episiotomy, between the vagina and rectum, is kept scrupulously clean. You will continue to have a heavy vaginal discharge (lochia), which gradually subsides during the first month at home. Originally blood-tinged, this discharge gradually becomes more and more yellowish and eventually disappears. Once the secretion is light enough and the perineum has healed sufficiently, you may use a tampon instead of an external pad. You can use a tampon anytime after a cesarean section, if it is agreeable with your physician. If you nurse, you may have a clear vaginal discharge for a longer period of time and, of course, may not have periods. In the event of a sudden heavy increase in the amount of blood in your lochia, call your doctor. Generally speaking, you will have your first menstrual period (provided you are not nursing) somewhere during the first four to eight weeks after delivery. It is all right to use birth control pills as a form of contraception if you are not nursing. You may begin them while you are in the hospital.

Medications

Continue to take your vitamin supplements for several months after you deliver, and if you are nursing, take the supplement until your baby is weaned. You may require no other medication except an occasional laxative. However, if you need something for pain or for the blues, your doctor will order it for you.

Sex and the New Mother

Generally speaking, before you have been home too long, *somebody* will think of sex again, and suddenly a great amount of activity and interest is generated in that direction. Although your episiotomy will have healed within a few weeks, there is often enough residual discomfort to make vaginal penetration uncomfortable. It is a good idea to avoid this degree of sexual activity until after your first office visit, but not many people do! Remember, though, you may be fertile and you do not want to make your first postpartum visit your first prenatal visit. You may make love without vaginal penetration anytime you want to.

Postpartum Check

While you are still in the hospital after delivery, it is a good idea to call your doctor's office and make arrangements for your first postpartum examination, which should be about six weeks after you leave the hospital. By then you are recovered sufficiently so that the doctor can examine you thoroughly to make sure that your body has healed and the uterus is back to normal size, shape, and position. Also at this time you want to discuss with him the various methods of birth control, provided you plan to avoid populating the world. The alternatives are presented to you in the next section. If a Pap smear is due, it will be taken at that time; if not, the doctor will be able to tell you when you must return for it. This is probably the most important single test a woman has available to her today. If for no other reason than obtaining your Pap smear, a postpartum visit is of fundamental importance because it continues and reinforces the concept of a regular checkup. If you have any trouble with your breasts or if you are nursing, your doctor may want to examine your breasts, as he undoubtedly will during your annual checkup.

Returning to the Workaday World

In today's environment you will probably want to—probably have to—return to your former employment. Most organizations now have specific maternity leave policies, and generally you can return to work with your position and seniority intact. The average leave time is six weeks after the actual date of delivery. If there have been complications of the pregnancy or delivery, or if a cesarean section has taken place, then six weeks may not suffice. Moreover, if your baby has been ill, even with something as simple as colic, you may have had little rest and little time to devote to your own life and affairs. Under any of these circumstances, you should ask your doctor for a statement to your employer explaining the problems and asking for extended recovery time. Usually this is granted, but you may be asked to consult with a company doctor as well. No matter. Be sure you are ready to return when you do return.

Here are some further points about working after delivery.

- It is generally good for you to get back to your work environment, particularly if you enjoy what you do and the people you work with. It gets you out of the house and prevents cabin fever. Moreover, it is very important that you keep your own life going, and this is a good, rewarding way to start.
- It is obvious that some jobs are more physical than others. Thus a forklift operator, a forest ranger, a secretary, a floor duty nurse, and a commercial airline pilot all must meet different requirements before returning to their duties after childbirth.
- Many studies show that the separation from your child is not in the least detrimental to your relationship with each other or to the child's emotional growth and security—all provided, of course, that you do spend quality time together and continue to bond.
- You are now fulfilling many roles: parent, partner, worker, housekeeper, cook, and lover. This is a difficult assignment, and you will need and deserve help from that other partner in order for all roles to be fulfilled. Thus if it's Saturday night at 11 o'clock and you have had a rough week at the office (worker), and an aggressive, active fussy, child all day (parent), and in the meantime did the week's laundry (housekeeper) and the weekend's menu (cook), you don't have much reserve left if the call to arms should come (lover, partner). So share the wealth and the work.

It is increasingly important in your own personal life to be able to plan adequately for the growth and development of your family. At this point you or your partner or both may begin to equate self-control with birth control. To this end, you may want to familiarize yourself with the most common acceptable forms of personal family planning.

More Children?

The Pill

The original oral contraceptive was a sleeping pill. As time went on, this was replaced by the Late, Late Show, which was even less effective. Neither offered 24-hour protection, and lots of normal healthy people make love at other times than bedtime. The market was there, and so in the early 1950s there became available "the pill" itself—the *real* pill—a combination of hormones that resemble female hormones and have the unfailing ability to prevent ovulation. They provided, therefore, almost 100 percent protection. True, they have occasional side effects, which may include weight gain, retention of fluid, depression, changes in sexual desire, suppression of menstrual flow, headaches, visual disturbances, changes in coagulation of the blood, leg cramps, and more. But most of these side effects are reversible when use of the pill is discontinued. Intravascular clotting with pulmonary embolism and death, so often heard about, is *exceedingly* rare. A relationship between the pill and cancer has never been truly established, but there is a suspicion that the pill *may* be related to the development of some very rare liver cancers. Balancing that risk, however, is newfound evidence that women who have been on oral contraceptives for some time have a significant decrease in the rate of development of ovarian cancer.

We believe that the pill should not be used after you reach the middle thirties, because there is a potential relationship between oral contraceptives and heart disease in middle age. If you smoke, this relationship increases *fortyfold!* It is also important to know that you should not take oral contraceptives for more than two consecutive years without a rest interval. Neither should you conceive until you have been off the pill for three or four months.

Absence of menstruation may occur when you get off the pill, and it is sometimes very difficult to treat. No menstruation means no conception. Most of the pill's complications are less deadly and less serious than the risks of pregnancy and much less so than many other things we do. However, pregnancy may soon be safer than any contraceptive. But if we rearranged our lives on the basis of risks involved, we would have to stop the following, on the basis of statistics alone, before stopping birth control pills: smoking cigarettes; drinking alcohol; driving cars and boats; flying; swimming; taking tub baths; sunbathing; becoming pregnant; downing aspirin, iron, sedative, pain, or diet pills; and so on. They are *all* more dangerous than the pill.

The IUD

Some people feel that if you're not taking pills you are simply taking chances. However, there are a number of plastic or metal intrauterine devices—IUDs—that can be inserted into the uterus and left there, and that are very effective methods of birth control—almost as effective as the pill. No one really knows for sure how these gadgets work, but it is assumed they prevent the implantation of fertilized ova in the uterine wall. Such devices are usually inserted before the end of a menstrual flow, and sometimes this insertion produces significant discomfort. They are difficult to place in women who have not had children, but it can be done.

IUDs are not 100 percent effective. Of pregnancies that do take place, most occur in the first year after insertion. The rate of pregnancy is around 2 percent at first, decreasing each year thereafter. Occasionally it is necessary to remove an IUD because of side effects, such as prolonged and heavy bleeding both during and between periods, severe cramping, or recurrent infection. A plastic IUD may be left in place indefinitely if there are no local reactions. The new copper and/or hormone IUDs must be replaced every few years.

The Rest

None of the other contraceptive devices compare in preventing pregnancy to the pill or the IUD. Diaphragms, jellies, creams, foams, condoms (rubbers, sheaths, safes) are reasonably effective if they are used conscientiously. Often, at the hearth of passion or in the heat of battle, they are forgotten.

Nursing is nature's way of contraception. Generally a nursing mother will not ovulate, and the longer she nurses, the longer she is unable to conceive. This is why, generations ago, women nursed until they could no longer stand the bites inflicted on their nipples by their "babies." However, ovulation *can* occur during nursing and so, therefore, can pregnancy.

Speed Breeding

Those of you who are interested in populating the world and increasing our risks of imminent extinction, plan your birth control in this general area. We include here rhythm, withdrawal, douches, and hunches.

Male Sterilization

Permanent and virtually perfect birth control is achieved by ligation of either the male vas deferens or the female fallopian tubes. Let's consider first ligation of the vas.

Advantages:

- It can be done anytime, providing the operating physician is satisfied that his or her patient is a responsible adult able to give his informed consent and wanting no more children.
- It is a relatively safe, simple, quick procedure that can be done under local anesthesia. Vas ligation is, therefore, usually an office procedure with only a few days' disability.

- It has no proved long- or short-term effects—except sterilization. Read on, though.
- Its effectiveness is very easy to prove: A negative sperm count indicates success.

Disadvantages:

- It is permanent. True, microsurgery can reconnect the tubes, but it is not always successful, and when vas ligation is done, it should be assumed that it is to be permanent. Is that a disadvantage? It is if you change your mind or your partner later in life.
- Other than the possible complications of any minor surgery, there are two side effects that need mentioning. There is some evidence that after vas ligation, immune changes may occur which, in some men, can hasten the onset of arteriosclerosis (hardening of the arteries). Further, the act of sterilization rarely may induce psychological changes resulting in impotence, at least temporarily.

Female Sterilization

Bilateral tubal ligation has become a relatively simple procedure to arrange for and to accomplish. There are few legal or medical obstacles left to performing this minor surgery on mature consenting women.

Frequently the tubes are tied through a very small incision immediately after delivery. If delivery is by cesarean section, then of course there is no need for any further incision. The tubes can be clipped, tied, sectioned, or removed; it makes little difference how they are interrupted. Having your tubes tied at delivery usually requires that you spend no longer in the hospital than you normally would. There are some situations, however, that make immediate tubal ligation unsafe after a vaginal delivery. Your doctor knows this and may put off surgery for

24–48 hours after delivery, or may even elect to do it some months later. This latter situation is known as an interval sterilization.

Elective interval sterilization is now a relatively simple procedure commonly done without hospital admission, that is, as an outpatient. You are given a light general or local anesthetic, and a small hollow tube is inserted into your abdomen just below your navel. Your fallopian tubes are easily seen and localized and are then crushed, cauterized, or pulled through a small plastic ring and pinched off completely. After a few hours of recovery, you go home. Very rarely, something can go wrong with this seemingly simple procedure, as it can with any operation. Therefore, you might, however unlikely it is, end up with a big incision in your abdomen and several days in the hospital.

There is another type of interval sterilization performed nowadays called a minilap tubal ligation. This procedure avoids some of the problems associated with the umbilical type of procedure and is done through a small incision slightly below the pubic hairline. Each fallopian tube is grasped and a portion removed therefrom. This separates the ends completely from each other.

Here are some things to think about, for and against ligation.

Advantages:

- It eliminates the need for birth control pills or any other devices.
- It is a permanent sterilization.
- It is almost foolproof.
- It has no sexual or other side effects that can be directly attributed to the procedure.
- It is relatively simple and very safe.

Disadvantages:

- It is permanent. Here again there are microsurgical techniques to reverse tubal ligation, but this surgery is not always successful. So tubal ligation should be considered a permanent sterilization procedure.
- Fallopian tube ligation is not as simple as ligating the vas in a male.
- It is usually more expensive than a vas ligation (unless you have comprehensive insurance). Your insurance may not cover the procedure at all. You had better check first.

Fascinating Facts

▷ Ten million women take the pill and 2,307,000 wear an IUD; 4,500,000 do something else, but over 3,000,000 women practice no birth control at all!

▷ Following are some facts and figures worth pondering. Some of them have been presented in earlier sections of your book. They are worth bringing together here. The figures are derived from many sources and are as accurate as such statistics can be. Your conclusions, if any, are your own and they are as good as anyone else's. But think.

U.S.A.

	Deliveries	In Hospital	Section Percent	Maternal Deaths	Fetal Deaths	World Population
1940	2,500,000	56%	3	9,300 (1 in 30)	117,500 (1 in 21)	2,300,000,000
1980	3,500,000	99%	16.5	245 (1 in 14,000)	43,400 (1 in 80)	4,309,000,000

1980   Legal abortions in the United States—1,200,000

269

DIARY

My Tenth Month

At last!

My Thoughts and Feelings

_____

_____

_____

_____

_____

_____

_____

_____

_____

_____

_____

_____

_____

_____

_____

_____

_____

_____

_____

_____

_____

_____

MY TENTH LUNAR MONTH

APPENDIX: OBSTETRICAL TECHNOLOGY

Obstetrical technology is growing at an incredible pace. This Appendix is devoted to a brief encounter with most of the new techniques, tests, devices, and procedures that share in the present-day delivery of obstetrical care. Your own doctor will be aware when and how these programs change, and throughout your book you will see how they apply to specific obstetrical problems.

Genetics

All of us have been endowed with a genetic code that clothes us with our unalterable, inherited characteristics. Of all the magic and mystery that enshroud procreation and life, none surpasses the binding of the total and absolutely necessary coded material into a single sperm head and a single ovum, which then unite with each other to unravel that fantastic code and weave, on an embryo's magic loom, a new body, mind, and spirit with the characteristics—good, bad, and indifferent—of both parents and a heavenly host of ancestors and progenitors.

Geneticists found that in each human cell there are forty-six chromosomes—twenty-two pairs of autosomes and two sex chromosomes. Women have two X sex chromosomes (XX) and men an X and a Y sex chromosome (XY). Now then, the female's two Xs actually outweigh the male's XY, and also carry more information. Let me point out, however, that most often, of the female's two Xs, only one is working; the other is lying

273

at the bottom of each cell, apparently doing nothing. We can see this phenomenon under the microscope. The nonworking X chromosome is called a Barr body (after the scientist who discovered the phenomenon); its presence (or absence) helps us in the study of certain genetic and infertility problems.

Of the forty-six paired chromosomes in each cell, one member of each pair comes from the sperm, one from the ovum. (The split of the paired chromosomes occurs just as the egg and sperm mature.) Since half of the sperm contain X sex chromosomes and half contain Y, and since all ova contain only one X, then it follows that the male determines the sex.

Each chromosome contains a number of stations or dots, called genes, and these, too, are paired: some genes are "dominant" and some "recessive," and recessives "give" to the dominant gene. Thus, brown eyes (*BB*) dominate blue eyes (*bb*), and a union of these two traits would always produce a brown-eyed child (anyway, almost always). Although oversimplified, that is basically the principle involved in dominant and recessive genes and their function.

Chromosomes—and genes—can be damaged by X rays, toxic substances, heat (but not cold, so embryos can be frozen), age, and certain other conditions. Most defective embryos are detected by nature and aborted spontaneously. Those that elude the natural scanning process can be identified by amniocentesis. Genetic counseling and amniocentesis are entered into when:

- There is a familial or racial history of an inherited disorder.
- The couple involved have already had a genetically abnormal child.
- The chance of an abnormal genetic pattern is high, as with a mother in her forties.

Genetic counselors are specialists who can advise expectant parents of their chances of passing on any inherited traits that either of them may carry in their own chromosomes. Such specialists also interpret the harvest from amniocentesis cultures and can give absolute advice on the genetic well-being of a developing fetus.

Amniocentesis

Amniotic Fluid

The fetus is enclosed in two sacs, the more proximate one being called the amniotic sac or membrane. Within its confines, besides the fetus, is a clear liquid appropriately called the amniotic fluid, which increases from 80 cc (2¾ oz.) at twelve weeks to as much as 1500 cc (1½ quarts) at term. Too much fluid (hydramnios) or too little (oligohydramnios) may occur, and such extremes usually, but not always, signify a fetal disturbance or a structural abnormality.

Water, which accounts for 98 percent of the fluid, is renewed about every 3 hours, while other components (electrolytes, proteins, etc.) change at a slower pace. This renewal phenomenon indicates that an amniotic circulation must exist, and indeed it does, although the mechanism is not altogether clear. A term infant swallows about 450 cc of amniotic fluid every 24 hours and quite regularly empties its bladder back into the amniotic sac. But these basic exchanges are insufficient to account for the total renewal of all amniotic elements. Other maternal-fetal circulatory and exchange mechanisms are obviously involved, but as yet they are not completely understood.

Amniotic fluid serves to protect the fetus by providing constant temperature and pressure, plus a shock-absorbing environment that allows free body movement and growth. There are undoubtedly many other amniotic fluid functions that are unknown. The fluid also contains some fetal debris, traces of meconium (a forerunner of stools) from the rectum, and lanugo (soft downy body hair), as well as surface fetal skin cells that regularly fall away as new skin cells come from below. Finally there are chemical substances circulating in the amniotic fluid. These substances are under constant study, and some are now used in a variety of tests to indicate fetal well-being, growth, and development, and to help identify certain inherited problems such as sickle cell anemia.

Genetic Analysis Early in Pregnancy

As the word indicates, *amniocentesis* is the removal of amniotic fluid from the amniotic sac. For our purposes this is almost always accomplished by means of a transabdominal (through the maternal skin, abdominal wall, and uterus) needle puncture. There are several particular times in pregnancy that this procedure is brought into use for analysis.

If there is a possibility of an inherited or age-related disorder that could affect the fetus, amniocentesis is resorted to at the fifteenth week of pregnancy or closely thereabouts. Carefully guided by ultrasound, and under local anesthesia, a needle is inserted through the abdomen and uterus into the amniotic sac, and a measured amount of fluid is withdrawn. Some of this is used for certain chemical tests (alpha fetoprotein, or AFP, test, for instance, which determines closure of the spinal canal, see p. 280), and is more accurate than the usual blood test. Most of the fluid, however, ends up being cultured so that the fetal skin cells within it may grow and be harvested in two or three weeks. (Such cell growth rarely fails, but it can, and a repeat amniocentesis may be necessary.) The growing cells are finally harvested, and after chemical treatment to enlarge the nucleus, are photographed and the chromosomes identified within the large nucleus. Now a geneticist can review the chromosomes under a high-power microscope and identify abnormalities, if any exist. Chromosomal analysis is exceedingly accurate; it also allows, whether needed or not, the absolute prediction of the fetal sex.

You may well wonder why the fifteenth week is usually

chosen to initiate amniocentesis. Well, any earlier would not be likely to yield sufficient fluid for testing, and any later would make therapeutic abortion, if indicated by the analysis, a difficult procedure both emotionally and technically by the time results were in. The results obtained are used in genetic counseling with the expectant parents.

Risks of Early Amniocentesis

- *Failure.* There are a number of reasons for this:
    Insufficient amniotic fluid will prevent the operator from either establishing contact with the amniotic sac or withdrawing enough fluid for analysis.
    The placenta may be directly in the way and prevent entrance into the amniotic sac.
    Maternal obesity may prevent needle penetration of sufficient depth into the abdomen.
- *Spontaneous abortion.* Although miscarriage does follow some amniocentesis procedures, the rate of occurrence is less than 1 percent—a lower figure than one would expect in a similar population of pregnant women not having *any* procedure done at all.
- *Rh sensitization.* Minute amounts of fetal blood *may* escape into the maternal circulation. In certain cases a very few number of fetal red blood cells can produce an Rh interaction in the blood of its mother, provided that she is Rh negative and the fetus Rh positive. Since the fetal blood type is unknown, all Rh negative women are immediately vaccinated with the Rh immune globulin after amniocentesis and are revaccinated with the same Rh vaccine at 28 weeks. Again, this is done even though the fetal Rh type is still unknown. There are no serious risks in giving the vaccine, but there are real risks in not giving it.

Important Facts About Amniocentesis

- The reports that you anxiously await are generally available in three to four weeks, and you are contacted immediately.
- The costs at this writing vary in different locations across the United States from $700 to $1,000; the procedure is often covered by insurance. In some countries (Canada, for example) the national health plan will pick up the tab.
- The accuracy is virtually 100 percent, and genetic abnormality discovered is 3 to 5 percent of the pregnancies tested.
- Genetic counseling can be found at all tertiary maternity care centers (see p. 290) and in certain other locations. Your doctor is familiar with the center closest to you.

Other Reasons for Amniocentesis

The removal of amniotic fluid from around the baby becomes progressively easier as pregnancy advances (because there is more of it), and it has been found of great value in later pregnancy for:

- Evaluation of fetal lung maturity. There are many reasons why lung maturity is an important piece of information to generate before contemplating an early delivery. Amniotic fluid reveals evidence of this in a variety of biochemical tests.
- The determination of fetal well-being. In circumstances in which a child approaching term may be in jeopardy, such as if the mother has diabetes, if intrauterine growth retardation (IUGR) is suspected, or in Rh incompatibility, amniotic fluid is a key source of information in the establishment of fetal well-being or not so well-being.
- Premature rupture of the membrane (PROM). In the event that rupture may have taken place and cannot be simply detected by other means, the insertion of dye into the

278

amniotic fluid will help to determine the integrity of the fetal sac. Dye found later in the vagina is proof of rupture.
• Culturing. When the doctor suspects that an infection has developed in the fetal amniotic sac, fluid can be withdrawn for culturing purposes.

Chorionic Villi Sampling

This very new experimental technique, which is used to assist in the prenatal diagnosis of genetic and other developmental abnormalities, had its origins in China, Russia, Italy, and, lately, England. It is used in this country at one or two centers only, which have received special approval from the National Institute of Health. The technique involves sampling the chorionic villi, the fetal tissues eventually destined to make up the placenta and which also produce a positive pregnancy test (see chapter 1). Chorionic villi cover most of the fetal membranes in early pregnancy and, since they extend into the uterine cavity, can be removed by very discrete sampling through the cervical canal. The villi, being fetal in origin, yield to genetic analysis just as the amniotic fluid components do. At this time there are three methods used to obtain such samples.

• *Directional.* A hollow instrument, which allows one to see the fetal membranes and therefore the chorionic villi, is inserted through the cervix under direct visualization.
• *Blind.* A probe is inserted by touch alone through the cervix to sample the chorionic villi without direct visualization.
• *Ultrasound guide.* In this technique, real-time ultrasound is used to direct instrumentation and sampling.

Advantages

• The procedure can be done very early in pregnancy, which means less delay in diagnosis and easier termination of the pregnancy if it should be indicated.

- It is less hazardous than other techniques, in that when it works properly, the amniotic sac is not invaded.

Disadvantages

- Being an experimental procedure, it is not approved for general use anywhere in our country.
- Failure to succeed in obtaining sufficient sampling from around the embryo sometimes occurs.
- Embryo damage or destruction sometimes occurs.
- Accidental sampling of maternal tissues with false results sometimes occurs.

What Is Achieved

- Chromosomal analysis from the chorionic tissue, which is, of course, strictly fetal (unless contaminated with maternal tissue, as noted).
- DNA analysis. Techniques are now available for actually analyzing the DNA structure of the unborn infant to determine, among other things, presence of certain blood disorders. Since you are wondering, DNA (deoxyribonucleic acid) is the actual coded material making up the genes and chromosomes, which in turn order and control all growth, development, and body functions.

Alpha Fetoprotein Test (AFP)

This test, which you now know is routinely done in early amniocentesis procedures, can also be performed, with less precision, on maternal blood at about fourteen or fifteen weeks of pregnancy. By that time AFP should have almost disappeared from the fetal and therefore the maternal circulation, since the fetal neural tube and the spinal canal should be closed, and this is where the fluid originates. Obstetricians are just beginning to perform this test routinely in the office as acceptable test kits become available. Blood is taken from the mother's vein, and generally if the tests show AFP present in abnormal amounts in the maternal blood, an ultrasound is advised to determine the complete integrity and closure of the fetal spinal canal. This particular AFP procedure, then, is on its way to becoming a routine test in all pregnancies at about the fifteenth week.

Very low values of the AFP test in early pregnancy *may* indicate the presence of Downs syndrome, recent evidence has shown.

Ultrasound

The effect of the advent of present-day reliable ultrasound techniques in obstetrics is equivalent to the effect of the advent of the automobile or electricity on American society and economy around the turn of the century. It is difficult to comprehend the magnitude of the obstetrical information this procedure has spawned. Ultrasound provides us with very reliable, detailed data on what is going on inside the uterus, from the earliest days of pregnancy to the moment of delivery. Moreover, it is a device that is safe, practical, and almost universally available.

What is ultrasound? As the name implies, it is simply sound waves that are machine generated at a frequency so high that one cannot hear them. These small, very high frequency waves can penetrate into the body, bounce back from the more dense organs inside, and create an image for us to see on a screen.

Generally speaking, *real-time* ultrasound is used most often now in obstetrical examinations. Real time means that what you see on the screen is actually what is going on right then. Although what is on the screen is not frozen into a photo, photos can be made at any point and be preserved.

Further, ultrasound waves reflected from the tissues within the uterus can generate a picture that can be computer enhanced for even more detailed study.

Here are some examples of the use of ultrasound in obstetrics:

- Monitoring of the fetal heart. The fetal heart can be seen beating beginning at the seventh to eighth week of pregnancy. The absence of a heartbeat much after this time generally indicates serious fetal problems. So if the examination is repeated a few days or a week later and still no heart activity is seen, we generally consider this fact to be absolute evidence of fetal demise. This information is of real value both to mother and to doctor. It prevents the prolonged agonizing wait we often used to have for a sure sign that something had gone wrong. So while it is extremely rare and discouraging not to have a visible heartbeat by at least the ninth week, it is extremely reassuring to see it.
- Confirmation of the actual duration of pregnancy. Measurement of the fetal crown/rump length during the first three months of pregnancy gives, with an accuracy of plus or minus *four* days, the date of conception! After the first three months, measurement of the head size (biparietal diameter), the abdominal circumference, and the length of a femur (long leg bone) will reveal the same significant information. In later pregnancy two ultrasound examinations six weeks apart can also provide a very accurate assessment of fetal age. Knowing the true duration of pregnancy is of great importance in some risk situations in which an early delivery is indicated. Further, accurate dating determines once and for all when pregnancy is *actually, truly* going overdue. This knowledge has significant clinical as well as social importance.
- Estimating the fetal weight, using a variety of measurements, to within a few ounces of actual weight.
- Determination of the development of intrauterine growth retardation (IUGR). This condition may develop in a number of abnormal obstetrical circumstances, usually after the twenty-eighth week. It may be due to fetal damage from many sources in early pregnancy or to failure of placental function in later pregnancy from a number of disorders. IUGR is a very important obstetrical complication, and is

discussed further on pages 155–156.

- Identification of multiple pregnancies. Twins, triplets, and further are identified almost absolutely by ultrasound. Note, though, that "twins" are sometimes seen on early ultrasound examination, only to have one of them disappear a little later because one represents a false fetal sac. This is very new information. It is possible that as many as half of all pregnancies start out *appearing* as twins. So when an early ultrasound picture suggests twins, it needs to be repeated later.
- Investigation of abnormal bleeding in late pregnancy and even in early pregnancy, to locate the area of placental implantation or to locate other sources of abnormal bleeding.
- Identifying, locating, and documenting the presence and location of an intrauterine contraceptive device (IUD).
- Establishing fetal age and well-being. Prior to attempting certain surgical procedures to close the cervix in some types of recurrent premature labor, the fetal well-being and age need to be established very definitely. This is accomplished by ultrasound.
- Determination of the potential for causing harm and the nature of certain pelvic tumors and cysts of the reproductive organs. Ultrasound examination can assist in defining the characteristics of these growths and their potential for interfering with pregnancy.
- Identifying fetal abnormalities and disorders. Gross abnormalities and nowadays even small structural defects are being delineated by ultrasound.
- Determining the biophysical profile. Advanced ultrasound (level 2) analysis of fetal activity is being introduced in more and more obstetrical services throughout our country. Such analysis, carried out by highly skilled sonographers, measures many variables in the intrauterine environment and is reported in scores of 1 to 10 as a biophysical profile (BPP). Included are many fetal measurements, amniotic fluid volume, placental age, fetal breathing and movement activity such as hand

grasping, and more. The result of all this data is a very accurate assessment of fetal well-being. Its use is generally reserved for the last trimester of pregnancy in managing high-risk situations. It may well be that this biophysical profile (BPP) will replace stress and nonstress testing in the future.

- Determination of sex. The high resolution obtained in modern ultrasound can determine, with fair accuracy, the sex of the fetus. This is confined to last-trimester ultrasound procedures and is not considered an important diagnostic yield.

Risk

There are hundreds and hundreds of thousands of ultrasound pictures taken each year during pregnancy. Some authorities and experts have suggested the possibility that there may be some harm from all this piercing sound (like the effect of a soprano's C above high C in a test-tube fertility clinic!). While it is true, of course, that there is as yet no long-term follow-up of these children past fourteen years, there now exists no reliable evidence that any fetal or maternal damage is done by any ultrasound technique. I would suspect that such evidence would have surfaced by this time if there were any. One has, however, only to harken back to the DES crisis to caution against making broad-sweeping statements early on in any medical setting.

Fetal Monitor Systems

Physicians have always been vitally interested in and taken great store in intrauterine fetal activity, in particular the beating fetal heart. In the past we used stethoscopes to listen for fetal activity and fetal heartbeat. Even before that, as a listening device, we rolled up pieces of stout paper, such as you now find lining shirts as they come from the laundry—if your laundry still does that. By putting one end to our ear and the other on your tummy, we could hear an abundance of fetal activity. Some casual or more daring physicians in the past directly applied their ear to Madam's abdomen, and it would yield the same information—even more clearly. Today, however, most external monitoring is done with ultrasound devices that emit a very high wave length resembling closely those instruments used by submarines trying to detect what lies ahead, beside, or behind. Ultrasound waves are bounced back from the moving heart valves, and this is translated into an audible beat that can be clearly heard by both mother and physician—a very delightful sensation indeed.

Often this heartbeat is heard as early as the tenth week of pregnancy, depending on some variable factors that have nothing to do with the well-being of the child, such as the thickness of the mother's abdomen and the position of the uterus. The heart has actually been beating from about the seventh week. Anyway, these devices are used at each visit to listen for the fetal heart rate and sometimes for certain other things, such as the placenta location.

As pregnancy progresses, the heart rate becomes of more and more critical interest and value. There are many things going on inside that affect the maternal-fetal environment and that are reflected by the fetal heart rate. This is particularly true in infants being stressed by an internal environment that does not deliver enough food, oxygen, or both on a regular basis. Although great placental reserves are present to protect the fetus, certain conditions, such as chronic malnutrition, diabetes, high blood pressure, chronic alcohol and tobacco poisoning, and many other problems can obliterate such placental reserves as time and injury go on. Signs of reserve depletion usually appear after the twenty-eighth week, and the development of techniques to monitor and interpret heart rate values beyond this point has become a science unto itself.

There are a number of tests for placental reserve. The first that we have to consider is the Non-Stress Test (NST).

Non-Stress Test

First of all, some definitions: *fetal stress* means that something is going on in the fetal environment that is stressing the fetus in some way. The stress could be caused by an aging placenta, maternal illness such as diabetes, maternal starvation, or social poisoning (from alcohol or tobacco, for example)—any number of things. The infant reacts to such stress in several ways, one of which is reflected in its heart rate.

Stress is not necessarily damaging, any more than stress is to adults—to a certain point. Repeated and continued stress, however, can lead to *fetal distress.* In this situation the stress has continued and/or increased to a point at which the fetus is now in some real jeopardy, and intervention may be required.

A non-stress test attempts to measure fetal well-being without adding to any other stress that may already be affecting the fetus. This procedure can be done in the labor suite or in your doctor's office. An external ultrasound monitor is placed over the abdomen in the fetal heart area, and heartbeats are recorded on a monitoring strip of paper. This paper recording is the only thing that differs from the regular heart monitor that the doctor has already used to listen to the baby.

It is now known that under normal circumstances fetal heart activity varies with periods of wakefulness and sleep. These episodes occur at regular intervals. In a healthy pregnancy, the heart rate increases during periods of fetal activity at measured intervals. When this normal reaction is observed, we have a *reactive NST.* It indicates that the fetus is at present under no stress. On the other hand, failure of the heartbeat to speed up indicates a potential fetal problem and is designated a *nonreactive*

NST. Such tests are repeated every few days or weekly, depending on the circumstances and indications, but if they become nonreactive, we move on.

Fetal Stress Test

This procedure actually puts a certain amount of stress on the placenta and, therefore, the baby, and determines by so doing if fetal distress is present or imminent. This is the procedure to be followed if the NST becomes nonreactive, and its purpose is to indicate the possibility that some nutrient or oxygen supply problem may exist in the fetal environment.

In order to produce stress, the uterus is made to contract, much as it would in labor. To do this, we must start an intravenous infusion and administer oxytocin, a drug used to accelerate or induce labor. Further, now we add to the monitoring devices a gauge to determine the duration and amplitude of our induced uterine contractions. Under healthy circumstances, the fetal heart rate does not vary with a normal and customary uterine contraction. If, however, it is being deprived and therefore distressed during a contraction, the heartbeat changes and we have a positive oxytocin challenge test (OCT) or fetal stress test (FST). Either designation—OCT or FST—means the same thing. Any positive challenge test becomes a signal for an immediate full-scale review of the pregnancy.

Breast Stimulation Test

A new type of stress test is being investigated in this country and elsewhere. It is called the breast stimulation stress test (BST). We know that stimulation of the nipple produces uterine contractions by making a natural oxytocin substance appear in maternal blood; that's why afterpains are sharper while you nurse. We can, therefore, achieve the same results as the standard challenge test but without having to start an intravenous and without running the slight risk of excessive uterine contractions from the oxytocin medication. This simplified breast stimulation test (BST) is still under investigation and is not yet widely used.

Biophysical Profile

Finally, as we shall see, a level-two ultrasound examination yields us a biophysical profile (BPP) in late pregnancy—a test that may replace the NST and the OCT. (See Ultrasound, p. 281.)

Monitoring Labor and Delivery

In normal as well as abnormal labor, the monitoring equipment just described is used almost routinely to observe fetal heart rate and maternal uterine contraction activity. Thus we have a pretty reliable indicator of the child's well-being during labor and delivery as well as a record of maternal uterine activity while labor is progressing. The fetal heart rate pattern shows accelerations and decelerations under a variety of labor conditions, and these recorded observations are of significant value in protecting and guarding fetal well-being during the critical labor and delivery period.

Arguments are being raised against monitoring during normal labor, and some statistics have shown that it may be harmful and may, without cause, increase the rate of cesarean section operations. The overwhelming weight of evidence, however, is that monitoring during labor and delivery is of significant and protective value. Don't avoid it.

Fetoscopy and Fetal Surgery

With the advent of all the new techniques of evaluating fetal health and activity within the uterus, it became a challenge to see if we could extend our diagnostic arm even further and perhaps extend a therapeutic arm along with it. As a result, there is a brand-new specialty—fetology. This specialty, as the title indicates, is the study of unborn babies. There are few fetologists in this country and very few centers where fetology and its operative extensions, fetoscopy and fetal surgery, can be undertaken. *Fetoscopy* is a technique whereby the uterus is entered and the fetus observed directly with a fiberoptic lighted lens and a grasping apparatus, often equipped with the capability of taking certain samples. The fetoscope usually is inserted through the mother's abdomen and womb. This direct visualization allows for the detection of certain types of structural defects. The samples that are obtained consist of:

- Blood taken from the placental vessels. This is used to help determine certain types of blood disorders, such as sickle-cell anemia and thalassemia.
- Skin biopsies, removed to evaluate certain types of genetic skin disorders and used in genetic analysis.
- Muscle biopsies, taken to detect certain forms of cerebral palsy.

Fetoscopy Risks

The maternal risks are slight. Infection may occur, but this is unusual. Fetal risk consists of a 5 percent chance that premature labor and, as a consequence, death, may follow. These risks must be weighed carefully against the derived benefits.

Fetal Surgery

For the past several years fetal surgery has been performed by some fetologists. These techniques have been developed in order to try to save some unborn infants with problems that might otherwise make their survival out of the uterus impossible. As an example, hydrocephalus, a condition in which the head is very, very large, prevents normal delivery and also may, by the pressure of the fluid within the skull, destroy brain tissue. Therefore, techniques have been devised to reduce this pressure, divert the fluid from within the head, and allow the child to proceed to full term and delivery.

Another disorder that can be treated in the uterus results from congenital obstruction of the bladder and therefore leads to the backing up of urine in the kidneys, the destruction of the kidneys, and, by further stretching of the abdominal cavity, pressure atrophy of the abdominal wall muscles. Intrauterine surgery can divert the flow of urine directly into the amniotic sac, which is where fetal urine ends up anyway. This preserves the kidneys and, of course, the abdominal wall.

In order to do fetoscopy and fetal surgery it is mandatory to have:

- a tertiary care facility (see below) with all the technical expertise and equipment that this involves
- skilled fetology specialists
- superb ultrasound techniques
- good clinical skills in using labor-inhibiting drugs, so as to prevent uterine contractions and premature expulsion of the infant under study

Progress in fetology and fetal surgery is slow, and in some areas fetal surgery is almost at a standstill while the benefits and risks are being reevaluated.

Perinatal (Tertiary Care) Centers

In order to deliver maternal health care in the most effective possible way and at the least possible cost, doctors have instituted a nationwide network of perinatal centers. At the hub of each center is a class-three maternity unit. These tertiary centers, as they are also known, can manage the most critical obstetrical problems. The staff is skilled in maternal-fetal medicine, special infant care (neonatology), and obstetrical anesthesia. Further, all laboratory and support equipment this type of service may require, such as level-two ultrasound, is readily available.

In the communities surrounding each tertiary care center there are many secondary and primary obstetrical hospitals. A primary care hospital usually manages normal obstetrical patients. Secondary hospitals, on the other hand, are involved in the management of some complicated obstetrical problems, and their doctors perform operative procedures. Serious and dangerous complications, however, are referred up the chain to the tertiary care center. Thus, doctors practicing even in very remote areas of our country know that there is a big brother always ready and available to assist them and their mothers with major problems. Ambulances and helicopters are an integral part of each network.

As an example, the University of Tennessee Medical Center in Memphis is the tertiary care center for western Tennessee, eastern Arkansas, and northern Mississippi. If you look at a regional map you will see why this makes geographic sense. Almost every corner of the United States is thus organized to assure the very best obstetrical care in the world to American mothers.

If this is so, you may wonder why it is that the United States still rates about fourteenth in the world in fetal mortality. The answer to that is not to be found in the health care delivery system alone. It also lies in the diverse nature of our people, in our life-style, our dietary and social habits, and in our tremendous adolescent pregnancy population.

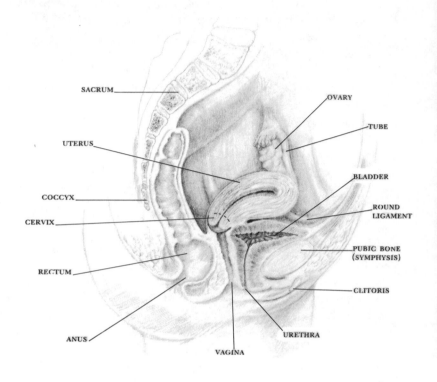

SACRUM

OVARY

TUBE

UTERUS

BLADDER

COCCYX

CERVIX

ROUND
LIGAMENT

PUBIC BONE
(SYMPHYSIS)

RECTUM

CLITORIS

ANUS

URETHRA

VAGINA

NORMAL ANATOMY

GLOSSARY

ABORTION   Loss of a pregnancy, either accidentally or purposefully, before viability (twenty-six weeks).

ACIDOSIS   A rare state of metabolic imbalance that may occur in diabetes, prolonged labor or in the *fetus* under certain circumstances, such as placental insufficiency.

AFP   See *Alpha Fetoprotein.*

AFTERBIRTH   A fetal structure attached to the uterine wall. See *placenta.*

ALBUMINURIA   Albumen (a protein) in the urine—an abnormal finding—often associated with kidney disorders and with *toxemia* of pregnancy.

ALPHA FETOPROTEIN (AFP)   A substance secreted by the *fetus* that becomes enclosed in its spinal canal system during early body development. Its presence in the maternal blood, and in the *amniotic fluid,* is used to indicate the health of the fetal spinal canal and cranial system.

AMNIOCENTESIS   Needle aspiration of *amniotic fluid* through the mother's abdomen for *chromosome* culture and many other tests.

AMNIOTIC FLUID   Liquid surrounding the *fetus,* composed of secretions from the *placenta,* fetal urine and other minor constituents. It circulates constantly and is replaced every few hours.

Note: Italicized words are defined elsewhere in the glossary.

ANALGESIA Relief of pain without loss of consciousness.

ANESTHESIA Complete relief of pain by either general or local agents; complete loss of consciousness in general.

ANTIBODIES Protein warriors formed by the body to defend against similar protein invaders; the basic principle of vaccination. May go astray in Rh disorders.

APGAR SCORE A method of rating a baby's condition at birth and five or more minutes later. It is the summation of a number of observed factors in the newborn, such as heart rate, respiratory rate, color, muscle activity, etc. A perfect score would be 10–10—rarely achieved.

AREOLA Pigmented skin area around breast nipples, which darkens during pregnancy. Montgomery follicles may appear in the areola, little raised white areas of no consequence.

AUTOSOMES Another name for *chromosomes,* excluding the sex chromosomes.

BABY BLUES See *depression.*

BARR BODY Females have two X *chromosomes,* but usually only one works. The other, which curls into a ball in the bottom of each cell's nucleus, is called a Barr body.

BETA HCG A highly specific fragment of the human *chorionic gonadotropin* (HCG) complex which is very important in assessing (1) the presence of pregnancy, (2) the health of the fetus, and (3) the diagnosis of an ectopic pregnancy.

BILIRUBIN Everybody has bilirubin in the blood, but an excess hemoglobin breakdown in newborns may produce excess bilirubin and jaundice—even without Rh disorders. The excess is generally treated by exposure to light, rarely by exchange transfusion.

BIOPHYSICAL PROFILE (BPP) A relatively new test for fetal well-being done in an *ultrasound* laboratory. Five different fetal conditions and activities are measured to achieve the final score. The test is usually done after the twenty-eighth week and is often repeated as term approaches. Also called fetal biophysical profile (FBP).

BONDING The psychological union of the mother, father, and child at the time of birth at that point when they first all touch, see, hear, and feel one another. It is most desireable immediately after birth, but there are some excellent alternatives if this cannot be done.

BPP See *biophysical profile.*

BRAXTON HICKS CONTRACTIONS Usually painless, sometimes painful, usually irregular, sometimes regular *contractions* of the uterus. They begin early in pregnancy and continue throughout, helping to force blood through the uterus.

BREAST STIMULATION TEST A relatively safe, noninvasive method of determining fetal well-being in the last trimester. Stimulation of the mother's nipple produces uterine *contractions,* and concurrent monitoring of the fetal heart rate indicates the baby's reaction to the stress of such a contraction.

BREECH A not uncommon presentation of a baby, in which the bottom instead of the head comes forth first.

CANDIDA ALBICANS Commonest cause of yeast infections in the vagina; likely to occur in pregnancy.

CATHETER A plastic or rubber tube to draw urine from the bladder. May be left in place (in-dwelling) for several days if necessary.

CAUDAL A form of *epidural anesthetic* administered very low in the epidural space.

CAUTERIZATION Electro-coagulation of infected tissue—usually cervical tissue—to produce healing.

CERVICAL OS The muscular fibrous ring that keeps the uterus closed until *labor* begins.

CERVIX Neck of the womb (*uterus*); the opening of the uterus into the back of the vagina.

CESAREAN SECTION Delivery of the baby through an abdominal incision rather than the normal vaginal route.

CHLOASMA Darkening of areas of the skin during pregnancy—e.g., breast areola, forehead, cheeks and abdomen.

CHORIONIC GONADOTROPIN The hormone of pregnancy secreted by the *placenta*, which produces the first positive evidence of pregnancy.

CHORIONIC SAMPLING A very new method of determining the genetic makeup of an *embryo*. Through the *cervix*, by a variety of techniques, direct samples are taken of the chorion, the fetal tissue which will form the *placenta*. This procedure can be done very early in pregnancy (at seven weeks). The samples are then analyzed genetically to determine the presence, or absence, of inherited disorders.

CHROMOSOME Each cell has twenty-three pairs of chromosomes. They carry the *genes*, which carry all the inherited characteristics.

CLASTOGEN A drug or substance that can damage a *fetus* without necessarily producing a visible defect.

COLOSTRUM The forerunner of milk, present in the breast as early as the second month.

CONCEPTION The union of a ripe ovum with a sperm to form a new life.

CONDYLOMATA ACCUMINATA A virus infection that produces innocuous warts at the entrance of the vagina, which sometimes extend into the vagina itself.

CONTRACTION STRESS TEST (CST) See *fetal stress test.*

CONTRACTION (UTERINE) The uterus contracts throughout most of pregnancy, generally with painless *Braxton Hicks contractions*. Sometimes such contractions are regular and produce false labor. But when labor begins, contractions become progressively closer and harder and are designed to evacuate the uterus of your baby.

CORPUS LUTEUM CYST A normal ovarian cyst that forms each month on the ovary at the point where ovulation occurs. Grows for the first three months of pregnancy, supporting the pregnancy, then disappears. May cause some pain in early pregnancy.

COUVADE SYNDROME The sharing of the symptoms of early pregnancy by the husband.

CPD Cephalo-pelvic disproportion, which exists when the presenting part or parts of the baby do not fit the pelvic bones and tissue structure.

CST See *fetal stress test.*

CYTOMEGALOVIRUS This rare virus can cause certain problems related to infertility and birth defects.

DELIVERY The act of expulsion of the baby, either through the vagina or through a *cesarean section* incision.

DEPRESSION A feeling of helplessness and hopelessness that can involve anyone at any time. It may occur during early pregnancy and soon after delivery, but is usually temporary unless there is an undercurrent of previous depression.

DIAPHRAGM A fairly effective birth control device. See also *diaphragmatic hernia.*

DIAPHRAGMATIC HERNIA A hiatus or epigastric hernia. Stomach tissue is pushed into the chest through the muscular diaphragm which separates the chest from the abdomen. Often occurs temporarily in late pregnancy.

DILATION The degree of openness of the *cervix,* which, usually closed till labor begins, dilates from one to ten centimeters during labor.

DIURETIC A medication that removes water from the body; usually not indicated in pregnancy except under certain conditions.

DIZYGOTIC TWINS Fraternal twins; two babies from two separate eggs.

DOWNS SYNDROME (MONGOLISM) A genetic birth defect, sometimes sporadic, sometimes inherited, much more common in babies of mothers over thirty-five. It is due to a translocation (abnormal location) of certain genes.

ECTOPIC PREGNANCY A pregnancy that implants anywhere outside the uterus; it may be in a *fallopian tube,* in an ovary, or even in the abdomen.

EDC Expected date of confinement, or delivery. Give or take a week or two.

EDEMA   Swelling of the tissues due to the retention of fluid.

ELECTROCYTES   Dissolved salts, buffering acids or alkalis normally found in the blood plasma or tissue fluids.

EMBRYO   A living human being that results from *conception* and if it remains in place leads to one of us.

EPIDURAL ANESTHETIC   Contrary to a *spinal block*, an epidural doesn't enter the spinal canal, but blocks nerve impulses as they leave the spinal canal. It has few side effects and usually offers the best type of pain relief for labor. A *caudal* is a particular form of epidural anesthetic.

EPIGASTRIC HERNIA   See *diaphragmatic hernia.*

EPISIOTOMY   An incision made in the *perineum* to prevent tears in the area or in the rectum and surrounding tissues.

FALLOPIAN TUBES   The tubes that conduct eggs to the uterus. Fertilization usually occurs in the tubes.

FBP   See *biophysical profile.*

FETAL BIOPHYSICAL PROFILE (FBP)   See *biophysical profile.*

FETAL MONITORS   Electronic devices which, when attached by proper leads and sensing devices on the mother's abdominal wall, measure uterine *contractions* and fetal heart rate during labor. At some point in *labor,* when the *cervix* is sufficiently dilated, the fetal sensor may be applied directly to the fetal scalp. Moreover, sometimes direct internal measurements of uterine contraction activity is possible by placing a very soft sensor high into the uterus—again through the opened cervix. Most labors in the United States are monitored. Fetal electronic monitors are also an integral part of the *fetal stress test* (FST), as well as the *nonstress test* (NST).

FETAL STRESS TEST (FST)   A procedure to determine the presence of fetal stress or distress in late pregnancy. Using intravenous pitocin, uterine *contractions* are produced and the fetal heart rate response to such contractions is measured and interpreted. This particular test is also known as a contraction stress test (CST) or as an oxytocin challenge test (OCT).

FETOLOGY   The study of unborn infants in their intrauterine environment.

FETOSCOPY   A relatively new science which studies the *fetus* and its uterine environment by a variety of invasive and noninvasive methods.

FETUS   An unborn child.

FORCEPS   Safe tonglike instruments used to extract babies late in labor. Occasionally used to turn babies lying in abnormal positions.

FST   See *fetal stress test.*

GENES   Ultra structures that are present on *chromosome* strands and control inherited characteristics.

GERMAN MEASLES (RUBELLA)   A simple virus disease which is of little significance unless it occurs during pregnancy. In early pregnancy, in particular, it can cause marked birth defects.

GRAVIDA   The number of times pregnancy has occurred or existed in any one patient—e.g., gravida 10 means ten conceptions, regardless of the outcome.

HCG   Human *chorionic gonadotropin.*

HERPES VIRUS II   A highly communicable venereal disease that is as yet without cure. Although its greatest danger for women is that it may be involved in the development of cancer of the *cervix,* it also has a known obstetrical fetal risk: Should there be an open herpes ulcer on the cervix, in the vagina, or on the vaginal entrance at the time of delivery, a *cesarean section* should be performed to safeguard the child from the possibility of developing systemic herpes after it passes through the birth canal.

HIATUS HERNIA   See *diaphragmatic hernia.*

HYALINE MEMBRANE DISEASE   Coating of fetal lungs which prevents adequate oxygen exchange. More common in premature infants, after cesarean section, and in some other obstetrical conditions. Also called respiratory distress syndrome.

HYDRAMNIOS   Excess amounts of *amniotic fluid* surrounding the baby, which may mean nothing or signify fetal defects.

HYPERTENSION   Elevation of resting blood pressure levels above normal limits—high blood pressure.

HYPERTENSION OF PREGNANCY   Formerly known as toxemia or pre-eclampsia and eclampsia, this condition, peculiar to human pregnancy, is characterized by *hypertension, edema,* and protein in the urine mainly in the last trimester.

INDUCTION OF LABOR   The artifical initiation of labor for any reason.

IUD   Intrauterine device: a plastic, metallic, or hormonal device inserted into the uterus for birth control.

LABOR   Productive uterine contractions which produce dilation of the cervix, descent of the baby and its expulsion into the world.

LA LÊCHE LEAGUE   A national group of individuals devoted to the encouragement of breast-feeding.

LAMAZE METHOD   An obstetrical learning method which prepares mothers and their husbands for the labor experience.

LANUGO   Downy soft hair that coats the body of immature babies.

LEBOYER METHOD   A quiet, peaceful delivery experience designed to reduce birth trauma to infants.

LECITHIN   A substance present in high ratios when fetal lungs are mature.

LIGHTENING   The baby drops into your pelvis and you can breathe again. Usually taking place in the last month of pregnancy, it may happen suddenly (a few hours) or over a period of days.

LOCHIA   Vaginal secretions of blood and fluids that persist after delivery on and off till the first menstrual flow. Never heavier than a menstrual flow or excessively irritating.

MISCARRIAGE   Accidental abortion.

MONGOLISM   See *Downs syndrome.*

MONOZYGOTIC TWINS Identical twins, coming from one ovum or egg.

MORNING SICKNESS Half of you will have it moderately, a few severely, during the first few months. It consists of nausea and/or vomiting, usually most bothersome in the early morning but sometimes lasting all day.

NEONATOLOGIST A pediatric specialist who takes care of distressed newborn babies.

NONSTRESS TEST (NST) This procedure is, at present, the most commonly used technique to assess fetal well-being during late pregnancy. A *fetus* with a normal central nervous system, unblunted by oxygen deprivation, moves about regularly within the *uterus*. Such movements are accompanied by accelerations of the fetal heart rate and, of course, the changing heart rate appears on a fetal monitoring device. Measurement of these basal heart rate changes therefore indicates the presence or absence of fetal distress. It is called a nonstress test because no uterine *contractions* are induced in the procedure such as are done in a *fetal stress test.*

NST See *nonstress test.*

OBSTETRICIAN A medical doctor who specializes in the handling of pregnancy and childbirth.

OCT See *fetal stress test.*

OVULATION The act of expulsion of an egg (ovum; pl., ova) from one ovary or the other.

OXYTOCIN A substance that can make the uterus contract either during *labor* or after delivery.

OXYTOCIN CHALLENGE TEST (OCT) See *fetal stress test.*

PAPANICOLAOU (PAP) SMEAR A very important annual test for protection against cancer of the *cervix.* It consists of a smear taken directly from the cervix and read by a trained technician.

PARA The number of full-term pregnancies sustained by any one mother.

PERINATOLOGY   A new science devoted to the identification and study of high-risk pregnancies as they approach and reach delivery.

PERINEUM   An anatomical area separating the vagina and the rectum.

PICA   The craving for unusual food—or nonfood—substances during pregnancy.

PLACENTA   The organ structure made by the *fetus* which invades its host (the mother) to a point and which performs tremendous hormone and metabolic functions during pregnancy. Also called afterbirth.

PLACENTAL BARRIER   A nebulous and probably nonexistent gate which supposedly keeps toxic substances away from a *fetus*.

PROGESTERONE   A very important pregnancy-related hormone excreted early in pregnancy by the *corpus luteum cyst* on the ovary and later by the placenta: it prevents expulsion of the fetus under ordinary circumstances.

PRONE PRESSURE SYNDROME   A feeling of weakness/faintness that often occurs when you lie on your back during pregnancy. Turn to your left side.

PROSTAGLANDINS   A group of newly discovered substances in our bodies that have profound effects on pregnancy as well as many other body systems.

PRURITUS OF PREGNANCY   A generalized body itching usually experienced in late pregnancy, which disappears after delivery. There may be no visible skin eruptions.

PTYALISM   The production of excess saliva during some pregnancies.

REGIONALIZED CARE   Almost all the U.S. is divided into regionalized perinatal centers. They are designated as follows: Level I indicates a delivery facility or hospital that is able to manage normal obstetrics. Level II units can manage normal obstetrics as well as cesarean sections and certain operative complications. Level III represents a highly sophisticated center that can respond to any obstetrical challenge. At the core is a level III unit that is surrounded by a number of class I and II units feeding in severe obstetrical and neonatal problems.

RELAXIN An anterior pituitary hormone which causes the ligaments in the pelvic girdle to soften and give during pregnancy. This makes *labor* easier and walking harder.

RH FACTOR A useless protein substance present in some 85 percent of us (Rh positive) and absent in the rest (Rh negative). It is of importance only in pregnancy and blood transfusions.

SADDLE BLOCK A form of *spinal block* anesthesia that involves only the very low abdomen and legs. It is useful for vaginal delivery.

SHOW A bloody/mucous vaginal discharge that occurs near the onset of labor.

SICKLE CELL ANEMIA A type of anemia found only in blacks, it may complicate pregnancy or vice versa.

SIDS Sudden infant death syndrome. There are many theories, but no solutions as yet. Also called crib death.

SITZ BATH A tender, soothing dunking of your bottom in warm water—ideally in a tub, but sometimes, in hospitals, a little plastic bowl must suffice.

SPINAL BLOCK Anesthesia that is accomplished by inserting a drug directly into the spinal fluid. May achieve any level of pain relief desired.

STRIAE When the belly expands, the skin over it stretches and produces the lines of striae, also called stretch marks.

TERATOGEN A drug or substance which can produce a physical abnormality in a *fetus*.

TETANIC UTERINE CONTRACTION A uterine *contraction* that lasts for a prolonged period of time—usually over one minute.

T. MYCOPLASMOSIS A rare vaginal infection that can interfere with fertility and reproduction.

TORCH This is a name given to a variety of infectious disorders that can have profound effects on a developing fetus (see chapter 4).

TOXEMIA "Poisoning of pregnancy," or pre-eclampsia, a condition found almost exclusively in the last third of human pregnancy, producing *edema, hypertension* and *albuminuria.* Becoming less and less common in our society. The condition is now called *hypertension of pregnancy.*

TOXOPLASMOSIS Cat fever, an infection of significance only in pregnant women. Usually transmitted by cats, but also by poorly cooked pork.

TRICHOMONAS A common, very irritating vaginal infection of no serious consequence.

ULTRASOUND Sound waves too high-pitched in frequency to be heard by us and having the ability to penetrate human tissues without radiation risk such as in X rays. Machines producing ultrasound waves are being used with increasing frequency in all medical areas today. Because of the safety factor, these machines are being widely used in obstetrical diagnostic procedures. Using them, we are able to determine the health, location, and duration of pregnancy and its growth and development as pregnancy advances. New uses for this invaluable tool are being reported each day. Recently the National Institutes of Health issued a series of ultrasound guidelines which stated that although years of experience with this device have revealed no harmful fetal effects, it still should not be used as a *routine* pregnancy testing tool.

ULTRASOUND LEVEL I, II Most *ultrasound* procedures are carried out with either the physician's own ultrasound equipment or as part of a regular radiology setting. This is level I technology. For more advanced analysis, a Level II ultrasound clinic is needed with highly sophisticated ultrasound equipment and physicians specially trained to interpret very precise, minute degrees of fetal growth, development, and well-being. Such clinics are part of a tertiary care obstetrical center and certain other specialized areas. See *regionalized care.*

UMBILICAL CORD   A cordlike fetal structure connecting baby and placenta. Twelve to thirty-six inches in length, it contains arteries which pump blood into the placenta and a vein which brings blood back to the infant.

UMBILICUS   Navel; belly button.

URETHRA   A short tube which connects the bladder to the outside world. Empties just above the vagina.

URINALYSIS   Routine urine testing for albumen, sugar, acetone, bacteria, pus and blood. Usually done each prenatal visit.

UTERUS   The womb; the reproductive organ that contains and nourishes a fetus until it is ready for expulsion—which is the uterus's climactic capability.

VERNIX CASEOSA   A white, cheesy, waxy substance which coats babies' skin in late pregnancy.

VIABLE   Able to survive; viability in babies usually is impossible before the twenty-eighth week of pregnancy.

WOMB   See *uterus*.

INDEX

ABOUT THE AUTHOR

Dr. Gillespie was born in Canada and received his medical degree from McGill University, Montreal. Most of his training in obstetrics and gynecology was done in the United States at Johns Hopkins and other teaching hospitals. He is certified by the American Board of Obstetrics and Gynecology, and is a Fellow of the American College of Obstetricians and Gynecologists. He was recently elected a Fellow of the Royal College of Obstetricians and Gynecologists in London, England. In his private practice in Little Rock, Arkansas, Dr. Gillespie specializes in high-risk obstetrics. He is also clinical professor of obstetrics and gynecology at the University of Arkansas School of Medicine.